Therapy of the Hand and Upper Extremity

Scott F.M. Duncan
Christopher W. Flowers

Therapy of the Hand and Upper Extremity

Rehabilitation Protocols

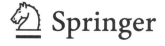 Springer

Scott F.M. Duncan
Department of Orthopedic
  Surgery
Boston University/Boston
  Medical Center
Boston, MA, USA

Christopher W. Flowers
Department of Orthopedic
  Surgery
Ochsner Medical Center
New Orleans, LA, USA

ISBN 978-3-319-14411-5   ISBN 978-3-319-14412-2   (eBook)
DOI 10.1007/978-3-319-14412-2

Library of Congress Control Number: 2015930049

Springer Cham Heidelberg New York Dordrecht London

Printed on acid-free paper

Springer International Publishing AG Switzerland
is part of Springer Science+Business Media (www.springer.com)

Preface

The purpose of this book is to provide the orthopedic surgeon and hand surgeon as well as the physical, occupational, and hand therapist with an easy, "go-to" quick reference source for potential rehabilitation protocols. By no means does this book represent the only way to rehabilitate an injury or a surgery postoperatively, but it does represent our collective synthesizing of various therapy protocols over the last 15 years. This book has been written to try and meet the need for a quick reference text for rehabilitative protocols that the active clinician needs in their practice.

The evolution of orthopedic surgery, hand surgery, and rehabilitative therapy has been challenging in that some treatments have not withstood the test of time or the rigors of scientific evaluation. Nonetheless, this book tries to still honor the art of medicine while incorporating the latest accepted rehabilitative protocols that many surgeons and therapists are currently using. No one protocol is necessarily entirely satisfactory, but these outlines of protocols should allow the surgeon and therapist to build upon them to meet the needs of their patients. One of the important aspects of rehabilitation is to understand the different phases of treatment and that not all phases are necessarily "cut and dry," ending at one particular point of time and beginning at another. Much of therapy is really a fluid situation and must be adjusted accordingly to the type of surgery (or injury) as well as the day-to-day condition of the patient. There is the old adage that great therapy can overcome even mediocre surgeries, and in some cases, that adage is quite correct. As therapy visits become more expensive for patients with higher deductibles and higher co-pays, as well as a limit on the absolute number of visits that the payer will cover, it is all the more important for each therapy visit to have a more significant impact both educationally as well as on the patient's physical condition.

In conclusion, we hope that this book benefits patients and helps the orthopedic surgeon, hand surgeon, physical therapist, occupational therapist, and the hand therapist provide better care for the patients that they all serve. We appreciate the many mentors who have imparted this knowledge to us, and this book represents our humble way of giving back for what so many have given to us.

Boston, MA   Scott F.M. Duncan
New Orleans, LA   Christopher W. Flowers

Contents

Part V   Elbow Sports Injuries

Part VI   Elbow Trauma

Part VII   Wrist Bone Injuries

Part IX   Wrist: Nerve Compression

Part X   Wrist Tendon Injuries

Part XI   Hand/Finger Bone Injuries

About the Authors

Scott F.M. Duncan M.D., M.P.H., M.B.A. is the Chair of Orthopedic Surgery at Boston University School of Medicine and Chief of Orthopedic Surgery at Boston Medical Center. Prior to this, he was System Chair of Orthopedic Surgery at Ochsner Health System. He received a Bachelor's Degree in Biology from Harvard University and went on to receive a Doctorate of Medicine from the University of Washington School of Medicine and a Master's Degree of Public Health in Epidemiology from the University of Washington School of Public Health. Dr. Duncan then completed an internship in general surgery at the University of Tennessee in Memphis and residency training in orthopedic surgery at the Campbell Clinic—University of Tennessee. He received his fellowship training in hand surgery, upper extremity surgery, and microsurgery at the Hospital for Special Surgery—Cornell Medical College in New York City. Dr. Duncan also has a Master's Degree of Business Administration in Healthcare from the University of Texas at Dallas.

Dr. Duncan worked at the Mayo Clinic in Arizona and the Mayo Clinic Health System in Minnesota for almost 10 years before joining Ochsner in 2011 and then Boston University in 2015. Dr. Duncan is board certified in orthopedic surgery by the American Board of Orthopedic Surgeons and has a Certificate of Added Qualifications in Hand Surgery.

Dr. Duncan has published numerous articles and book chapters on topics related to upper extremity surgery. He edited the textbook *Reoperative Hand Surgery* (Springer, 2012), which is utilized as a resource for hand surgeons worldwide for complex reoperative hand surgery cases. Dr. Duncan's clinical subspecialty practice involves hand, elbow, and shoulder surgery, as well as microsurgery.

Christopher W. Flowers M.D. received his Bachelors Degree from Morehouse College in Atlanta, Georgia in 2007 and went to The University of Texas Medical Branch at Galveston from 2007 to 2011 to receive his Doctorate of Medicine. He then completed his internship and began his residency at Ochsner Clinic Foundation in New Orleans, LA. His current post-residency plans involve applying for a Sports Medicine Fellowship. His research interests involve bridging the gap between the multiple teams involved in orthopedic patient care as well as various sports medicine related topics.

Part I
Shoulder Arthroplasty

Chapter 1
Hemiarthroplasty/Total Shoulder Arthroplasty

Sling × 3 weeks (with immobilizer), Continue sling for three more weeks as needed

1–2 Weeks

- Goals:
    - Minimize pain and inflammation
    - Achieve staged PROM goals (avoid aggressive PROM)
    - Maintain integrity of replaced joint
    - Scapular stabilization
    - No active shoulder ROM, lifting, supporting body weight or lifting of body weight with hands, AVOID any shoulder hyperextension

- Exercises Days 1–3:
    - Pendulum hangs
    - Finger, wrist, and elbow AROM (no weight) Maintain integrity of replaced joint
    - Shoulder PROM: 100° Flexion, gentle ER to 30°, IR to chest and 45° Abduction

- Exercises Days 3–10:
    - Continue PROM—flexion, abduction, ER as tolerated in the scapular plane
        - * NO Extension PROM, IR/ER in plane of scapula

S.F.M. Duncan and C.W. Flowers, *Therapy of the Hand and Upper Extremity: Rehabilitation Protocols*, DOI 10.1007/978-3-319-14412-2_1, © Springer International Publishing Switzerland 2015

- ○ Begin resisted hand, wrist, and elbow AROM
- ○ Resume general conditioning (walking, stationary bicycle)

    * NO Treadmill walking or elliptical

- ○ Begin scapular isometrics and submaximal shoulder isometrics (in neutral)
- ○ Pulleys (flexion and abduction)—as long as greater than 90° of PROM
- Exercises 10 Days–3 Weeks:

  - ○ Continue PROM progression as tolerated (NO hyperextension)—limiting ER to protect subscapularis reattachment.
  - ○ Gradually progress to shoulder AAROM.

Criteria before Phase 2: Shoulder PROM flexion/abd (90°), ER (45°), IR (70°), isometric activation of all shoulder musculature

3–6 Weeks

- Continue PROM progression, begin AROM
- Reestablish dynamic shoulder stability
- Continue PROM as tolerated, begin supine AROM flex/abd/IR/ER
- Begin AAROM horizontal adduction
- Begin rotator cuff and periscapular isometrics
- Begin scapular strengthening and stabilizations

Criteria before Phase 3: Supine shoulder PROM flexion (140°), abd (120°), ER (60°), IR (70°), elevate above 100° with good mechanics

6–12 Weeks

- Gradual restoration of shoulder strength, power, and endurance
- Optimize neuromuscular control
- Gradual return to functional activities with involved upper extremity

- Continue AROM as tolerated, begin IR/ER in scapular plane
- Begin gentle AAROM IR behind back
- Begin light functional activities
- Week 8: Begin progressive supine active elevation (anterior deltoid strengthening) with light weights (1–3 lb) and variable degrees of elevation
- Week 10: Begin resisted flexion, Abduction, ER (therabands/sport cords)
- Week 10: Progress IR behind back to AROM (AVOID overstretching)

Criteria before Phase 4: Supine shoulder PROM flexion (140°), abd (120°), ER (60°), IR (70°), elevate above 120° with good mechanics

12–24 Weeks

- Enhance functional use of upper extremity
- Improve muscular strength, power, and endurance
- Gradual return to advanced functional activities
- Gradually progress strengthening, add closed chain activities as tolerated
- Home exercise program 3–4 times per week
- Gradual return to moderately challenging functional activities

4–6 months — Return to recreational hobbies, gardening, sports, golf, doubles tennis

Chapter 2
Reverse Total Shoulder Arthroplasty

Sling × 3 weeks (with immobilizer), Continue sling as needed for three more weeks

1–3 Weeks

- Minimize pain and inflammation
- Achieve staged ROM goals (avoid aggressive PROM)
- Promote healing
- Scapular stabilization
- No active shoulder ROM, lifting, supporting body weight or lifting of body weight with hands
- Pendulum hangs
- AROM/AAROM: c-spine, elbow, wrist, and hand (no weight)
- Supine shoulder PROM: flexion/abd to 90° in the scapular plane, 20° ER (NO IR) being careful not to stress ER for subscapularis reattachment
- Begin periscapular/deltoid sub-maximal pain-free isometrics in the scapular plane

4–6 Weeks

- Supine shoulder PROM: flexion/abd as tolerated, ER as tolerated, IR to belt line
- No IR or extension, no lifting arm against gravity
- Begin gentle resisted exercises of elbow, wrist, and hand

S.F.M. Duncan and C.W. Flowers, *Therapy of the Hand and Upper Extremity: Rehabilitation Protocols*,
DOI 10.1007/978-3-319-14412-2_2,
© Springer International Publishing Switzerland 2015

- Begin rotator cuff strengthening and deltoid strengthening with gravity eliminated
- Progress scapula and trapezius work with light resistance

7–8 Weeks

- Progress pain-free PROM, begin AROM
- Continue to restrict hyperextension shoulder ROM
- Progress PROM as tolerated, begin PROM IR to tolerance ($<50°$) in the scapular plane
- Begin AAROM/AROM: progress from supine to sitting/ standing as tolerated (NO ext)
- Begin gentle glenohumeral IR and ER sub-maximal pain-free isometrics
- Begin gentle scapulothoracic rhythmic stabilizations and supine isometrics

9–12 Weeks

- Week 10: Begin standing-forward punch, seated rows, shrugs, bicep curls, and bear hugs
- Begin gentle periscapular and deltoid sub-maximal isotonic strengthening exercises
- Begin AROM with light resistance: supine flex/abd, side-lying IR/ER

12–16 Weeks

- Enhance functional use of operative extremity and advance functional activities
- Enhance shoulder mechanics, muscular strength, and endurance

    * NO lifting greater than 6 lb

- Progress to gentle standing resisted flex/abd

17+ Weeks

- Continue strength gains
- Maintenance/Home exercise program
- Home exercise program 3–4 times per week
- Progression toward a return to functional activities within limits per MD

Part II
Shoulder Sports Injuries

Chapter 3
AC Joint Reconstruction

Sling for 5 weeks

0–3 Weeks

- Minimize pain and inflammation
- Full elbow and wrist ROM
- Home exercise program
- Protect fixation from weight of arm or anything over 5 lb

    * AVOID elevation past 90° for first 4 weeks
    * AVOID excessive reaching and IR/ER for first 5 weeks

- Pendulums, ball squeezes
- Theraband triceps and biceps exercises
- Isometric rotator cuff IR/ER, shoulder Abd/Add, flex, ext with arm at side ONLY

4–7 Weeks

- Progressive shoulder ROM to 90° flexion/abduction
- Minimize pain/swelling
- Avoid stressing fixation
- Continue pendulums/PROM
- Begin supine ER and forward flexion to full as tolerated, begin IR to full as tolerated
- Week 6: Begin AROM with terminal stress to prescribed limits as tolerated

S.F.M. Duncan and C.W. Flowers, *Therapy of the Hand and Upper Extremity: Rehabilitation Protocols*, DOI 10.1007/978-3-319-14412-2_3, © Springer International Publishing Switzerland 2015

- Week 7: Begin standing-forward punches, seated rows, shoulder shrugs, bicep curls, and bear hugs

8–11 Weeks

- Minimize overhead activities
- Begin maximizing gentle ROM in all planes
- Begin manual mobilizations of soft tissue, GH, and scapulothoracic joints for ROM
- Begin stick ROM, shoulder pulleys, scapular stabilizations, and PNF patterns

12+ Weeks

- Progressive increases in strength and endurance
- Full ROM in all planes
- Begin return to sport-specific exercises
- Begin aggressive rotator cuff strengthening program
- Maximize ROM in all planes
- Increase strength and functional training for gradual return to activities
- Return to specific sports determined by PT and MD clearance

Golf: 3–4 months, Tennis: 4 months, Contact Sports: 4–5 months per MD clearance

Chapter 4
Arthroscopic Anterior Stabilization (Latarjet Procedure)

Sling with Abd pillow×6 weeks (with immobilizer—remove pillow at week 4)

For SLAP Repair—NO resisted Biceps×4 weeks

RESTRICTIONS—Avoid shoulder Extension and External Rotation during the first 6–8 weeks,

No EMPTY CAN throughout rehab under any circumstance

Phase I

- 1–3 Weeks:

  ○ Goals:

    – Minimize pain and inflammation
    – Promote healing and protect repair
    – Gradual increase in Passive ROM
    – Ensure adequate scapular function

  ○ Restrictions:

    – No Active ROM
    – No lifting objects or removing arm from sling
    – Avoid excessive external rotation as described above

  ○ Exercises:

    – Passive, Active-Assistive, and Active ROM of the elbow, wrist, and hand

S.F.M. Duncan and C.W. Flowers, *Therapy of the Hand and Upper Extremity: Rehabilitation Protocols*, DOI 10.1007/978-3-319-14412-2_4,
© Springer International Publishing Switzerland 2015

- Begin pain-free shoulder PASSIVE ROM

  * Forward Flexion as tolerated
  * Abduction in plane of scapula as tolerated
  * Internal Rotation to 45° (at 30° abduction ONLY)
  * External Rotation in the scapular plane 0–25°—
    Begin at 30–40° Abduction
  * Caution with ER, light and as tolerated as to not
    disrupt anterior capsule

- Scapular clock exercises with progression to scapular
  isometrics
- Ball squeezes
- *SLEEP*: add towel under elbow to prevent shoulder
  hyperextension
- Postural exercises

Phase II

- 4–9 Weeks:

  ○ Goals:

    - Minimize pain and inflammation
    - Protect integrity of repair
    - Gradually increase Active ROM
    - Gradually wean out of sling weeks 4–5 per MD
    - Begin light waist-level activities

  ○ Restrictions:

    - No Active ROM until adequate Passive ROM with
      good mechanics
    - No lifting of objects with affected arm
    - Avoid excessive external rotation as described above
    - No activities or exercises that place excessive load on
      the anterior capsule (push-ups, pec flys, etc.)
    - No scaption with internal rotation (empty can) dur-
      ing ANY stage of rehab

  ○ Exercises Weeks 4–5:

    - Progress shoulder PASSIVE ROM

      * Forward Flexion as tolerated

* Abduction in plane of scapula as tolerated
* Internal Rotation to 45° (at 30° abduction ONLY)
* External Rotation in the scapular plane 0–45° — Begin at 30–40° Abduction
* Caution with ER, light and as tolerated as to not disrupt anterior capsule
* All passive — (ONLY flexion and ER/IR (in scapular plane) AAROM)

- Glenohumeral joint mobilizations as indicated — if ROM restricted (Grade I, II Only) — only until desired ROM is reached
- Address scapulothoracic and trunk joint mobility (T-Spine joint mobilizations if needed Grades 1–3)
- Begin posterior capsular stretching as indicated (Cross-body adduction, Sleeper stretch)

○ Exercises Weeks 6–9:

- Progress shoulder PASSIVE ROM

  * Forward Flexion and Abduction in plane of scapula as tolerated
  * Internal Rotation as tolerated at multiple angles of abduction
  * External Rotation as tolerated — progress to multiple angles of abduction once ≥35° at 0–40° Abduction

- Glenohumeral joint mobilizations as indicated (Grade I–IV)
- Progress to AAROM/AROM with good mechanics
- Begin Rhythmic stabilization drills

  * ER/IR in the scapular plane
  * Flex/Ext and Abd/Add at various angles of elevation

- Continue AROM Elbow, Wrist, and Hand
- Strengthen scapular retractors and upward rotators
- Initiate balanced AROM/Strengthening program

  * Initially in low dynamic positions
  * Gain muscular endurance with high volume (30–50) Low resistance (1–3 lb)

* Full elevation in scapular plane before elevation in other planes
* Open and closed chain exercises
* NO heavy lifting or plyometrics at this time
* *Initiate**:
  * Full scapular plane raises to 90° with good mechanics
  * ER/IR strengthening with resistance tubing at 0° Abd using towel roll
  * Sidelying ER with towel roll
  * Manual resistance ER supine in scapular plane (light resistance)
  * Prone rows at 30/45/90° Abd to Neutral arm position

**Criteria before Phase 3: Passive forward elevation (115°), Passive external rotation (within 8–10° of contralateral side at 20° abduction), Passive external rotation at least 75° at 90° Abduction, Appropriate scapular posture at rest and dynamic scapular control with ROM and functional activities

Phase III

* 10–15 Weeks:
  * Goals:
    * Normalize strength, endurance, and neuromuscular control
    * Return to chest level full functional activities
    * Gradual and planned buildup of stress to anterior joint capsule
  * Restrictions:
    * Do not overstress the anterior capsule with aggressive overhead activities/strengthening
    * Avoid contact sports/activities
    * Do not perform strengthening or functional activities in a given plan until the patient has near full ROM and strength in that plane of movement

○ Exercises:

  – Continue Passive and Active ROM as indicated
  – Begin biceps curls with light resistance, progress as tolerated
  – Begin pectoralis major and minor strengthening—progress as tolerated

    * Avoid excessive stress to anterior capsule

  – Progress subscapularis strengthening (upper and lower)

    * Push up plus
    * Cross-body diagonals with resistive tubing
    * IR resistive band (0, 45, 90° Abduction)
    * Forward punch

**Criteria before Phase 4: Passive forward flexion WNL, Passive external rotation at all angles of abduction WNL, Active forward elevation WNL with good mechanics, Appropriate rotator cuff and scapular muscular performance for chest level activities*

Phase IV

• 16–20 Weeks:

  ○ Goals:

    – Continue stretching and PROM as needed/indicated
    – Maintain full non-painful AROM
    – Return to full non-painful AROM
    – Return to full recreational activities

  ○ Restrictions:

    – Avoid excessive anterior capsule stress
    – With weight lifting, avoid tricep dips, wide grip bench press, and no military press or lat pulls behind the head
    – Do not begin throwing or overhead athletics until cleared by MD (usually 4 months)

○ Exercises:

- Continue all exercises above, progress to isotonic strengthening
- Overhead strengthening if ROM and strength below 90° elevation is good
- Continue shoulder stretching and strengthening at least 4 times per week
- Progressive return to upper extremity weight lifting program emphasizing the larger/primary upper extremity muscles (start light weight and high reps)
- Push-ups with elbows not flexed past 90°
- Begin plyometrics/interval sports program if cleared by PT and MD

Chapter 5
Arthroscopic Bankart/SLAP Repair +/– Capsulorrhaphy

Sling with Abd pillow×6 weeks (with immobilizer—remove pillow at week 4)

1–2 Weeks

- Minimize pain and inflammation
- Promote healing and protect repair
- Gradual increase in ROM
- ROM limits to: Flexion (90°), Abduction (45°), ER−(20°), IR 30° in scapular plane, Extension—Neutral

  * All passive (ONLY flexion AAROM)
  * NO terminal stretching

- Begin pain-free submaximal isometrics in immobilizer (flex/ext/abd/add/IR/ER)
- Begin elbow, hand, and wrist exercises
- Pendulums with light weight
- Periscapular strengthening with manual resistance

3–4 Weeks

- Minimize pain and inflammation
- Enhance upper extremity strength
- Gradually increase ROM

S.F.M. Duncan and C.W. Flowers, *Therapy of the Hand and Upper Extremity: Rehabilitation Protocols*, DOI 10.1007/978-3-319-14412-2_5, © Springer International Publishing Switzerland 2015

- ROM limits to: Flexion (90°), Abduction (90°), ER—15° in scapular plane, IR 60° in scapular plane, Extension—15°

    * All passive—(ONLY flexion and ER/IR (in scapular plane) AAROM)

- Begin AAROM exercises standing or supine with wand/stick, wall walks

5–6 Weeks

- ROM limits to: Flexion as tolerated, Abduction as tolerated, ER—30° in scapular plane, IR as tolerated in scapular plane, Extension—30°

    * Begin AROM (Avoid active extension and ER past neutral)

- Advance IR to full, begin light theraband IR/ER exercises with elbow at neutral
- Begin UBE for endurance
- Begin supine rhythmic stabilizations at 90° flexion
- Prone strengthening—horizontal abduction (90° max), extension
- Begin flexion, scaption, empty can, and scapular strengthening (focus on eccentrics)

7–12 Weeks

- Minimize pain and inflammation
- Enhance upper extremity strength, endurance, and neuromuscular control
- Reach full ROM by week 10, normalize arthrokinematics
- Progress PROM as tolerated, begin gentle ER at 90° Abduction AAROM
- Begin plyo-toss chest passes at weeks 8–10
- Begin theraband PNF patterns and manual resistance supine PNF patterns
- Progress UBE for strengthening and endurance
- Begin isokinetic IR/ER at neutral at weeks 10–12

12–24 Weeks

- Full ROM
- Maximize upper extremity strength, endurance, and neuromuscular control
- Initiate sports-specific and functional training
- Begin posterior capsule stretching, towel stretching, and Grade 3/4 joint mobs PRN for full ROM
- Progress strengthening to increased resistance and high-speed repetitions
- Progress with eccentric strengthening of posterior cuff and scapular musculature
- Begin single-arm plyo-toss
- Progress rhythmic stabilization activities to include standing PNF patterns w/tubing
- Begin military press, bench press, and lat pulldowns
- Begin sport-specific drills and functional activities
- Begin interval throwing program at week 16
- Begin light plyometric program at week 12–16
- Progress isokinetics to 90° Abduction at high speeds

Chapter 6
Arthroscopic Posterior Labral Repair

Sling × 3 weeks (with immobilizer), Continue sling for three more weeks as needed

1–6 Weeks

- Goals:
    - Minimize pain and inflammation
    - Reestablish pain-free ROM
    - Protect repair
    - Improve neuromuscular control of the scapula in neutral GH position
- Exercises Week 1:
    - Forearm, wrist, and elbow PROM and active strengthening in all planes (isometrics, hand gripping)
    - PROM Shoulder (ONLY Passive) — Flexion/Abduction (60°), Extension (0°), IR/ER — perform only in 0–30° Abduction (ER to full as tolerated, IR to 0°)
- Exercises Weeks 2–4:
    - Continue shoulder PROM, begin gentle AAROM — All same as week 1, progress abduction to (90°)
    - Progress resistance/weight for wrist/hand/forearm/elbow

S.F.M. Duncan and C.W. Flowers, *Therapy of the Hand and Upper Extremity: Rehabilitation Protocols*,
DOI 10.1007/978-3-319-14412-2_6,
© Springer International Publishing Switzerland 2015

- ○ Begin Pendulums, overhead pulleys, table slides, and stick within ROM restrictions
- ○ Begin shoulder isometrics (sub-max, pain-free)—NO IR/ER
- Exercises Weeks 5–6:
  - ○ Initiate IR/ER Isometrics
  - ○ Begin scapulothoracic strengthening program
  - ○ Progress to AROM within ROM restrictions (may add resistance if pain-free—NO resistance for rotator cuff strengthening)
    - * ROM progression—Flexion (progress to full), extension/abduction/ER (full), IR from 0–30° Abduction (45°)

Criteria before Phase 2: Staged ROM goals achieved, minimal to no pain

7–9 Weeks

- Regain and improve upper extremity muscular strength
- Improve neuromuscular control of the upper extremity complex
- Normalize arthrokinematics of the shoulder in single planes of motion
- Progress and maintain all full AROM/PROM, Progress IR ROM to full
- Progress resistance on previous exercises
- Begin resisted rotator cuff strengthening at 0–60° Abduction as tolerated
  - * Avoid excessive IR
- Upper extremity cycle

Criteria before Phase 3: Full ROM with minimal pain, strengthening exercises with minimal pain

10–15 Weeks

- Near full rotator cuff strength
- Good tolerance to rotator cuff and ballistic activity

- Preparation for gradual return to functional activities and early throwing
- Begin more aggressive strengthening of the shoulder musculature (weight stations, free weights)
- Begin isokinetics for IR/ER (if available)—300–360°/s initially, progress to 180–300°/s as tolerated
- Progress rotator cuff strengthening to 90° abduction position
- Throwing athletes can begin Throwing Athlete Exercise Program

4–5 Months

- Prepare for full functional return
- Begin light upper extremity plyometrics program
- Functional activities including lifting and return to work activities
- Isokinetic test if available (at 180, 240, and 300°/s)
- Non-throwing athletes may return to full sports at this time per MD clearance
- Throwing athletes—begin Interval Throwing Program—need MD Clearance for return

Chapter 7
Arthroscopic Rotator Cuff Repair (Large/Massive)

Sling × 8 weeks (immobilizer INCLUDED) — *AVOID* Shoulder IR and Ext

1–7 Weeks

- Minimize pain and inflammation
- Protect repair, allow healing
- Pendulums (NO active movement), shoulder shrugs
- Elbow, wrist and hand AROM, and ball squeezes
- PROM forward elevation in scapular plane (supine to 90°) at physical therapy (one visit per week)

8–12 Weeks

- Discontinue sling
- Progress PROM goals to full in all planes
- Achieve PROM goals in ER at 20° and 90° abduction (full)
- Begin posterior capsule stretching
- Submaximal isometrics with elbow flexed to 90°
- Theraband scapular retractions, periscapular strengthening (low weight, high reps)
- Begin AAROM flexion and progress to AROM flexion

S.F.M. Duncan and C.W. Flowers, *Therapy of the Hand and Upper Extremity: Rehabilitation Protocols*, DOI 10.1007/978-3-319-14412-2_7, © Springer International Publishing Switzerland 2015

3–4 Months

- Achieve staged ROM goals
- Minimize pain
- Improve strength, endurance, and power
- Increase functional activities
- Full ROM in all planes
- Progress isometrics and periscapular strengthening program
- CKC exercises for dynamic scapular, deltoid, and cuff stability
- Begin light PNF D1, D2, and manual resistance for cuff/deltoid/scapula
- Begin theraband IR/ER strengthening and progressive serratus anterior strengthening
- Progress to isotonic dumbbell exercises of deltoid and supraspinatus (3 lb max)

  * Strengthening program should emphasize high reps, low weight (max twice daily)

5–6 Months

- Normalize strength, endurance, and power
- Return to full ADLs and recreational activities
- Stretching PRN
- Continue deltoid/cuff/scapula strengthening (5 lb max for isotonic)—progress below

  * Prone isotonic strengthening
  * Decreasing amounts of external stabilization provided to shoulder girdle
  * Integrate functional patterns
  * Increase speed of movements
  * Integrate kinesthetic awareness exercises into strengthening
  * Progress to decreased rest time to improve endurance

- Progress CKC dynamic stability activities
- Begin isokinetic strengthening

7–8 Months

- Stretching PRN
- Initiate plyometric program if warranted (2 hand tosses to 1 hand stability drills to 1 handed tosses—vary amount of abduction and protected ER)

    * Criteria: 5/5 MMT for cuff and scapula, begin program with light weight

- Continue deltoid/cuff/scapula strengthening program

Criteria before Return to Sports: MD Clearance, 5/5 MMT, complete plyometric program if warranted, complete interval return to sport program if warranted

Chapter 8
Arthroscopic Rotator Cuff Repair (Small/Medium)

Sling for 6 weeks (Sleep included)

1–6 Weeks

- Goals:
    - ○ Minimize pain and inflammation
    - ○ Achieve staged ROM goals (avoid aggressive PROM) Protect repair
    - ○ Protect repair
    - ○ Scapular stabilization
    - ○ Discontinue abduction pillow at 4 weeks, sling for 2 weeks following
    - ○ No active shoulder ROM, lifting, supporting body weight or lifting of body weight with hands

- Exercises Days 1–10:
    - ○ Pendulum hangs (NO active movement)
    - ○ Finger, wrist, and elbow AROM (no weight), Elbow PROM only if biceps tenodesis performed
    - ○ Begin seated scapular isometrics and cervical ROM
    - ○ Begin PROM flexion (60–90°) and ER @ 20° Abduction (0–15°)
        - * PROM in plane of scapula

S.F.M. Duncan and C.W. Flowers, *Therapy of the Hand and Upper Extremity: Rehabilitation Protocols*,
DOI 10.1007/978-3-319-14412-2_8,
© Springer International Publishing Switzerland 2015

- Exercises Weeks 2–3:
  - Continue PROM progression—flexion (60–100°) and ER @ 20° Abduction (0–20°)
    * No Internal Rotation or Extension PROM
  - Begin resisted finger, wrist, and elbow AROM
  - Resume general conditioning (walking, stationary bicycle)
    * NO Treadmill walking or elliptical
  - Begin manual scapular strengthening exercises
- Exercises Weeks 4–6:
  - Continue PROM progression—flexion (90–125°) and ER @ 20° Abduction (15–40°)
    * For Subscap repairs—ER at 0° Abduction (0–30°) PROM/AAROM for 6 weeks unless MD orders otherwise
  - Begin Joint mobilizations (Grades 1 and 2) for all shoulder joints as tolerated
  - Progress scapular isometrics as tolerated (sidelying retractions)
    * For Biceps Tenodesis—delay elbow flexion strengthening × 6 weeks
  - Avoid UBE

  Criteria before Phase 2: *Staged ROM goals achieved, minimal to no pain*

7–12 Weeks

- Allow soft tissue healing, don't overstress repair
- Gradually restore full PROM by week 12
- Minimize pain and inflammation
- RESTRICTIONS for Out of Sling:
  * No lifting anything heavier than a coffee cup for ADLs
  * No ROM beyond staged goals or excessive behind-the-back movements

* No supporting body weight with hands or arms
* No sudden jerking motions
* No long lever rotator cuff strengthening exercises that can stress repair
* No empty can exercises at ANY stage of rehab

- Begin gentle scapular/glenohumeral joint mobilizations to regain full PROM
- Progress from prone scapular retractions to prone rows to neutral extensions
- Begin PROM in other planes (horizontal adduction, ER @ 45°/70°/90° Abduction)
- Week 7: PROM flexion (120–140°), ER @ 20° Abduction (30–60°), ER @ 90° Abduction (40–60°)
- Week 9: PROM flexion (130–155°), ER @ 20° Abduction (45–60°+), ER @ 90° Abduction (50–75°), AROM flexion (80–120°)
- Week 7: AAROM as tolerated
- Week 10–12: AROM with focus on good mechanics; exercises:

  * Sidelying to supine to standing scaption, supine to side-lying ER with towel under arm as needed, supine pro-traction (progress from wand to without), push-up plus (progress from PWB on wall to table to weight bench to floor), prone rows, prone extension with ER, prone horizontal abduction with ER, prone scaption (week 9)

- When good mechanics and pain-free, initiate strengthening program for deltoid/non-repaired RC segments/scapula musculature

  * Light resistive band exercises in pain-free ROM, scapular strengthening program, low-level closed chain program

- Neuromuscular re-education—scapular mobility, core stability

Criteria before Phase 3: Staged ROM goals achieved with minimal pain, strengthening exercises with minimal pain, good static and dynamic posture

3–6 Months

- FULL Pain-free PROM/AROM
- Enhance dynamic shoulder stability and neuromuscular control
- Gradual restoration of shoulder strength and endurance
- Gradual return to full functional activities
- AVOID: lifting objects 15–20 lb, sudden lifting or jerking and overhead lifting
- Week 12: PROM flexion (140°–WNL), ER @ 20° Abduction (WNL), ER @ 90° Abduction (75°–WNL), AROM Flexion (115–145°+)
- Week 12: Begin functional IR stretch (behind the back)
- Begin light PNF diagonals for cuff/deltoid/scapula
- Begin open chain rhythmic stabilizations
- Begin closed chain activity progression
- Begin advanced strengthening program (ASP) as tolerated (Criteria for ASP: MMT at least 4/5, pain-free basic ADLs and initial strengthening program, full AROM elevation, goal is return to sports/heavy labor)

  * Sample ex: T-Band standing PNF, T-Band 90/90 ER/IR, T-Band sport simulations

Criteria before Phase 4: Adequate strength and dynamic stability for progression to higher demanding work/sport-specific activities

7+ Months

- Maintain full pain-free ROM
- Advanced conditioning, muscular strength, power, and endurance
- Begin return-to-sport training
- Continue strengthening progression to sport-specific programs (Throwers 10)
- Progressive return to weight-lifting program: begin light weight, high reps — progress to higher weight/lower reps
- Begin plyometrics program
- Initiate interval sport program after successful 3–6 week plyometric program

Criteria before Return to Work/Sports: MD Clearance, no pain at rest, minimal pain with activities, no sensation of instability, sufficient ROM for desired activities, adequate strength and endurance of RC and scapular musculature with minimal to no pain or difficulty

Chapter 9
Arthroscopic Subacromial Decompression, +/– Acromioplasty/Distal Clavicle Excision, +/– Biceps Tenotomy

Sling for 2 weeks

1–2 Weeks

- Minimize pain—Sling for 2 weeks comfort if needed
- Pain-free ROM (90° pain-free elevation)
- 4/5 MMT
- Focused arthrokinematics
- PROM/AAROM: t-bar, overhead pulleys, wall walks, shrugs
- Joint mobilizations (Grades 1–2)—GH, ST, AC, SC Joints
- Manual PNF for scapular stabilizers
- Capsular stretches (GENTLE)
- Submax isometrics, closed chain weight bearing, PRE for wrist and elbow

3–6 Weeks

- Minimize pain/Modalities
- FULL Pain-free ROM
- Increase to 5/5 MMT
- Normal arthrokinematics
- Progress previous exercises, continue joint mobilizations

S.F.M. Duncan and C.W. Flowers, *Therapy of the Hand and Upper Extremity: Rehabilitation Protocols*, DOI 10.1007/978-3-319-14412-2_9,

- Begin UBE, AROM, resisted flexion, scaption
- Scapular stabilization and rotator cuff PRE
- Begin bilateral Plyoball toss
- Core and trunk stabilization

7–12 Weeks

- FULL Pain-free ROM
- Isokinetic deficit <10 %
- Aggressive strengthening
- Emphasis on dynamic control and posterior cuff eccentrics
- Begin PNF diagonals, rotator cuff Plyoball, and plyometric progression
- Biodex IR/ER in neutral (180–300°/s)

13–16 Weeks

- Return to full activity
- Return to full sports activity via physician clearance
- Home program and discontinue formal PT

Chapter 10
Humeral Head Microfracture

Non-Weight Bearing 6 weeks to operative shoulder
  Sling 2–4 weeks for comfort

1–2 Weeks

- Minimize pain—Sling for comfort if needed
- Pain-free ROM (90° pain-free elevation)
- Focused arthrokinematics
- PROM: t-bar, overhead pulleys, shrugs (Progress to AAROM)
- CPM 6–8 h daily (IF REQUESTED)—90° abduction and ER, Begin Pendulums (800 per day beginning day 1 after surgery)
- Sub-max isometrics, PRE for wrist

3–6 Weeks

- Minimize pain/Modalities
- Increase pain-free ROM
- Progress previous exercises, continue joint mobilizations
- Begin AAROM/AROM in all directions, begin grade I/II GH distraction mobs
- Core and trunk stabilization (NO weight on arm/shoulder)

S.F.M. Duncan and C.W. Flowers, *Therapy of the Hand and Upper Extremity: Rehabilitation Protocols*, DOI 10.1007/978-3-319-14412-2_10,
© Springer International Publishing Switzerland 2015

7–12 Weeks

- FULL Pain-free ROM
- MMT 4/5 by week 12
- Begin light strengthening exercises (isometric IR/ER/scaption), PNF diagonals, periscapular strengthening, and postural focus
- Emphasis on dynamic control and posterior cuff eccentrics
- Begin lower extremity strengthening program to avoid atrophy
- Week 10: begin grade II/III GH joint distractions and inferior/posterior glides

13–16 Weeks

- Increase UE strength and endurance
- Begin PROM IR/ER at 90° abduction
- Progress strengthening exercises (unrestricted), begin plyometric progression

17+ Weeks

- Begin return to functional activity, begin weight-lifting regimen
- All activities allowed at 16 weeks, but overhead competitive athletics restricted for 6 months per MD clearance

Chapter 11
Pectoralis Major Repair

Sling with pillow × 6 weeks (immobilizer included)

1–2 Weeks

- Minimize pain and inflammation
- Maintain integrity of repair
- Gradually increase PROM
- Focused arthrokinematics
- Pendulum exercises 4 times daily (flexion, circles)
- Elbow/hand gripping and ROM exercises

3–6 Weeks

- Minimize pain and inflammation
- Allow soft tissue healing
- Increase PROM
- Begin resisted elbow/wrist exercises w/light dumbbell (<5 lb)—shoulder in neutral
- PROM forward flexion to 130° with arm adducted only
- Shoulder shrugs, scapular retraction without resistance

7–12 Weeks

- FULL Pain-free ROM
- Normal scapular kinesia
- Discontinue sling
- Gentle AROM in pain-free ROM, *NO PROM*

S.F.M. Duncan and C.W. Flowers, *Therapy of the Hand and Upper Extremity: Rehabilitation Protocols*, DOI 10.1007/978-3-319-14412-2_11, © Springer International Publishing Switzerland 2015

- Begin AAROM (pulleys, supine wand, wall climb)—
  Flexion >90°, Abduction and ER to tolerance, IR and
  extension (wand behind back)
- Periscapular strengthening program (no push-ups plus)
- Isometric exercises (*AVOID* adduction, IR, and horizontal
  adduction)

13–23 Weeks

- Maintain full pain-free ROM
- Enhance functional use of UE, gradual return to functional activity
- Improve muscular strength and power
- Begin pectoralis major strengthening (single arm pulleys
  and bands—adduction, horizontal adduction, IR, forward
  flexion)
- Begin rotator cuff strengthening, can progress periscapular program to add push-ups plus against wall

24+ Weeks

- Gradual return to strenuous work activities
- Gradual return to recreational sport activities
- Continue stretching if any motion restrictions
- Begin push-ups plus on floor
- Full activity at Week 36, *HIGH WEIGHT, LOW
  REPETITION BENCH PRESS DISCOURAGED
  INDEFINITELY*

Chapter 12
Scapular Dyskinesia (Periscapular and Rotator Cuff Strengthening)

Phase I REHAB (1–2 Weeks)

- Control pain and inflammation
- Independent in HEP
- Initiate muscular strength and endurance training without pain
- Posterior capsule, cross-body adduction, anterior chest wall, pec minor stretching program
- Soft tissue/joint mobilizations if indicated
- Begin basic periscapular strengthening and stabilization exercises: Seated press-ups, scapular clock, thumb tacks, standing wall rhythmic stabilizations

    * Maintain retracted scapulae bilaterally throughout exercises, maintain proper body mechanics and position — figure 8 clavicle collar if indicated

- Begin core strengthening/stability program

Phase II REHAB (3–7 Weeks)

- Minimize pain with all exercises
- Enhance upper extremity strength and endurance
- Normalize dynamic balance, proprioception, and coordination

S.F.M. Duncan and C.W. Flowers, *Therapy of the Hand and Upper Extremity: Rehabilitation Protocols*, DOI 10.1007/978-3-319-14412-2_12, © Springer International Publishing Switzerland 2015

- Preparation for return to functional activities
- Continue UE stretching program
- Progress periscapular strengthening exercises: horizontal abduction with theraband, TVAs, shoulder shrugs, rows with scapular pinch
- Begin CKC strengthening: wall push-up progression, modified prone push-ups, CKC axial load ball rolls in varying degrees of abduction, Wall Angels, isometric shoulder extensions
- Begin rotator cuff strengthening exercises: sidelying IR/ER, IR/ER with theraband at $0°$ and $90°$, empty can/full can, PNF patterns, prone horizontal abduction in neutral and ER
- Begin upper body ergometer below $90°$, progress slowly, only good mechanics established

  * Maintain retracted scapulae bilaterally throughout exercises, maintain proper body mechanics and position

Phase III REHAB (9+ Weeks)

- Upper extremity maintenance program
- Return to sport-specific activity
- Maintenance strengthening with increased weights
- Maintenance flexibility/stretching program
- Continue UBE with increasing resistance
- Begin upper extremity plyometrics program—ball trampoline tosses/catches, push-ups plus
- Sport- or work-specific rehabilitation

Part III
Shoulder Trauma

Chapter 13
Clavicle Fracture

Sling for 4–10 days (For Comfort Only)

0–1 Weeks

- Goals:
    - Minimize pain and inflammation
    - Full elbow and wrist ROM
    - Scapular stabilization
    - No active shoulder ROM, lifting, supporting body weight, or lifting of body weight with hands

- Exercises Days 1–10:
    - Pendulum SWINGS
    - Squeeze ball

2–4 Weeks

- Pendulums to warm up
- Active ROM with passive stretching
- Gentle pulley for shoulder
- Isometric scapular PNF

4–8 Weeks

- Pendulums to warm up and continue with phase 2
- Begin resistance exercises
- May begin lifting 5 lb (ONLY AFTER 6 WEEKS)

S.F.M. Duncan and C.W. Flowers, *Therapy of the Hand and Upper Extremity: Rehabilitation Protocols*,
DOI 10.1007/978-3-319-14412-2_13,
© Springer International Publishing Switzerland 2015

- May begin elliptical without active arm movement
- Continue NWB UE
- Mid-range motion of rotator cuff (ER and IR rotations)
- Active and light resistance exercises (through 75 % of ROM as patient's symptoms permit) without shoulder elevation and extreme end ROM
- Strive for progressive gains to active 90° of shoulder flexion and abduction
- Shrugs, seated rows, etc.

8–12 Weeks

- Maintain full pain-free ROM
- Increase manual mobilizations of soft tissue as well as GHJ and scapulothoracic jts for ROM
- No repeated heavy-resisted exercises or lifting until 3 months

Golf: 8 weeks, chip/putt only Tennis: 3 months Contact Sports: 4 months (per MD clearance)

Chapter 14
Mid-Shaft Humerus Fracture Nonoperative

0–2 Weeks

- Keep in stabilizing splint or brace.
- Start PROM and AROM to wrist and fingers.

2–8 Weeks

- Exchange to Sarmiento Brace. Have fitted snug enough to stabilize fracture but loose enough to avoid skin complications.
- Keep on Sarmiento continuously until fracture union.
- Begin shoulder pendulums, and elbow PROM and AROM.
- Continue PROM and AROM to wrist, hand, and fingers.

8–10 Weeks

- MD to verify union.
- Once union, begin PROM and AROM to shoulder.
- No aggressive stretching. Limit external rotation to neutral and internal rotation to chest.

10 Weeks

- Gradually increase ROM exercises and stretching tolerances. Stretch to threshold of pain but not beyond.

S.F.M. Duncan and C.W. Flowers, *Therapy of the Hand and Upper Extremity: Rehabilitation Protocols*, DOI 10.1007/978-3-319-14412-2_14, © Springer International Publishing Switzerland 2015

12 Weeks

- Begin stretching starting with isometric shoulder strengthening exercises with arm in adduction.
- Advance to shoulder resistance strengthening exercises.
- Advance ROM and strength as tolerated.
- Focus on returning to work or activity-related goals.

Chapter 15
Midshaft Humerus ORIF

Sling 4 weeks. Limit ER to neutral and IR to chest

0–4 Weeks

- Keep in Sling, except for therapy and bathing (after 2 weeks).
- Begin shoulder pendulums, and elbow/wrist/finger PROM and AROM.

4–8 Weeks

- Discontinue Sling.
- Gradually increase ROM exercises and stretching tolerances. Stretch to threshold of pain, not beyond.

8–12 Weeks

- MD to verify union.
- Begin stretching starting with isometric shoulder strengthening exercises with arm in adduction.
- Advance to shoulder resistance strengthening exercises.

12 Weeks

- Advance ROM and strength as tolerated.
- Focus on returning to work or activity-related goals. Patient may utilize hand for dressing, bathing, hygiene, and eating without resistance.

S.F.M. Duncan and C.W. Flowers, *Therapy of the Hand and Upper Extremity: Rehabilitation Protocols*, DOI 10.1007/978-3-319-14412-2_15,
© Springer International Publishing Switzerland 2015

8 Weeks

- D/C the web spacer.
- Progressive strengthening may be initiated beginning with a nerf ball and progressing to a hand exerciser. In many cases gently strengthening can begin at 6 weeks.
- Progressive resistive activities.

Discharge Criteria

- Patient will be independent in dressing, hygiene, eating, bathing, and progressive household activities.

Chapter 16
Proximal Humerus Fracture Nonoperative

Sling 3–6 weeks. Avoid IR/ER except when in therapy

0–10 Days: Early Passive Motion

- Pendulum exercises, passive forward flexion, passive external rotation. Begin AROM on the elbow, wrist, forearm, and hand.
- Shoulder elevation and retraction exercises are initiated.

10 Days–3 Weeks

- Pendulum active assist forward flexion, active assistive external rotation to 40° only if patients pain under control.

3–6 Weeks

- Pendulum exercises, active assistive forward flexion, abduction to 90°, active assistive hyperextension (6 weeks). Begin gentle strengthening exercises for the elbow, forearm, wrist, and hand.
- Begin weaning patient off sling.

4 Weeks

- Isometrics:
  - Internal rotation, external rotation, anterior deltoid, posterior deltoid, middle deltoid.

S.F.M. Duncan and C.W. Flowers, *Therapy of the Hand and Upper Extremity: Rehabilitation Protocols*,
DOI 10.1007/978-3-319-14412-2_16,
© Springer International Publishing Switzerland 2015

6–8 Weeks

- Active forward flexion-supine, active forward flexion with weights, supine, forward flexion-erect-with towel.

8 Weeks

- Resistive exercises, stretching.

 ***Note*: crepitus at the fracture site with ROM should be noted and *stopped* until the MD has been notified.

Discharge Criteria

- Patient will be able to comb hair, wash face, reach into shoulder-high cabinets.

Chapter 17
Proximal Humerus Fracture ORIF

Sling 4 weeks

0–2 Weeks: Early Passive Motion

- Pendulum exercises, passive forward flexion, passive external rotation. Begin AROM on the elbow, wrist, forearm, and hand.
- Shoulder elevation and retraction exercises are initiated.

2–4 Weeks

- Pendulum active assist forward flexion, active assistive external rotation to 40° only if patients pain under control.

4–6 Weeks

- Pendulum exercises, active assistive forward flexion, abduction to 90°, active assistive hyperextension (6 weeks). Begin gentle strengthening exercises for the elbow, forearm, wrist, and hand.
- Begin weaning patient off sling.

6–8 Weeks

- Isometrics:
  - Internal rotation, external rotation, anterior deltoid, posterior deltoid, middle deltoid.

S.F.M. Duncan and C.W. Flowers, *Therapy of the Hand and Upper Extremity: Rehabilitation Protocols*, DOI 10.1007/978-3-319-14412-2_17,

- Active forward flexion-supine, active forward flexion with weights, supine, forward flexion-erect-with towel.

8 Weeks

- Resistive exercises, stretching.

  ***Note*: Crepitus at the fracture site with ROM should be noted and *stopped* until the MD has been notified.

Discharge Criteria

- Patient will be able to comb hair, wash face, reach into shoulder-high cabinets.

Part IV
Elbow Nerve Injuries

Chapter 18
Cubital Tunnel In Situ Release

2 Weeks

- The bulky compressive dressing is removed and edema control measures are initiated as necessary.
- Active and passive ROM exercises are initiated to the elbow, forearm, and wrist for 10 min each hour.
- Scar massage with lotion and manual desensitization exercises are initiated.
- Patient should be independent in eating, self-care, and dressing.

6 Weeks

- Progressive strengthening exercises may be initiated to the elbow, wrist, and hand. Nirschl exercises are frequently initiated beginning with no weight and progressing up to 4 lb over the course of a 4- to 6-week period.
- Patient should be able to lift 16 oz of fluid and pull and push the door open.

Discharge Criteria

- Patient should be independent in all self-care, dressing, and light ADL activities.

S.F.M. Duncan and C.W. Flowers, *Therapy of the Hand and Upper Extremity: Rehabilitation Protocols*, DOI 10.1007/978-3-319-14412-2_18, © Springer International Publishing Switzerland 2015

Chapter 19
Cubital Tunnel Syndrome Nonoperative

0–3 Weeks

- An "elbow pad" is applied for continual wear.
- Avoid extreme elbow flexion and activities which may cause pressure to the ulnar nerve (inside of elbow).
- If having numbness or tingling at night, an anterior/volar elbow splint in approximately 45 of flexion may be applied to wear at night.

***May wear during day if symptoms persist.

3–6 Weeks

- Follow-up visit with surgeon. If the symptoms have resolved splinting is gradually decreased.
- Minimize pressure on the elbow, repetitive flexion/extension of the elbow, and prolonged flexion of the elbow.
- If symptoms improving with elbow pad and the static splint, then the conservative management is continued. If not, then surgical intervention may be considered.

Strengthening: Once asymptomatic and pain-free, a progressive strengthening program may be initiated such as the Nirschl exercises.

S.F.M. Duncan and C.W. Flowers, *Therapy of the Hand and Upper Extremity: Rehabilitation Protocols*, DOI 10.1007/978-3-319-14412-2_19, © Springer International Publishing Switzerland 2015

Discharge Criteria

- Able to demonstrate protection techniques.
- Initiate at least two visits for home program. If symptoms resolved, return for strengthening program.

Chapter 20
Cubital Tunnel with Anterior Transposition

2 Weeks

- The bulky compressive dressing is removed and a light compressive dressing and/or other edema control measures are initiated as necessary.
- Scar massage with lotion and manual desensitization exercises may be initiated.
- No ADLs are allowed with the postoperative upper extremity.

3 Weeks

- Active and passive ROM exercises may be initiated to the elbow, forearm, and wrist six times a day for 10-min sessions. With elbow extension it is important to perform only AROM in order to not interfere with the healing of the flexor pronator mass.
- Patient may begin light finger eating activities, use hand as assist in ADLs and use hand for bathing.

6 Weeks

- PROM exercises may be initiated to the elbow in extension.

S.F.M. Duncan and C.W. Flowers, *Therapy of the Hand and Upper Extremity: Rehabilitation Protocols*, DOI 10.1007/978-3-319-14412-2_20, © Springer International Publishing Switzerland 2015

- Patient can use hand for dressing ADLs with minimal resistance including: pulling socks on, pulling pants on, and reaching into a pocket.

6–8 Weeks

- Progressive strengthening may be initiated beginning with putty and a hand exerciser and gradually progressing to Nirschl exercises.

  ○ Initially, the Nirschl exercises are performed without weighted resistance. As resistance is initiated with the Nirschl exercises it is generally begun with a ½ lb weight and progressed to a maximum of 4 lb.

- Patient should be progressed in ADLs to pulling and pushing open doors lifting containers of 12–15 oz and progressing as tolerated.

Discharge Criteria

- Independent in all dressing, eating, and hygiene activities. Beginning use in light housekeeping activities progressing to moderate.

Chapter 21
Cubital Tunnel with Intramuscular Transposition

2 Weeks

- The bulky compressive long arm dressing is removed and edema control is initiated as necessary. It is not uncommon to require light compressive dressings (above the elbow to the wrist level) for an additional week to 10 days.
- AROM exercises may be initiated to the elbow, forearm, and wrist six times a day for 10 min sessions. In addition, PROM exercises may be initiated to the wrist and forearm along with passive flexion to the elbow. Passive extension of the elbow is not permitted until 6 weeks postoperation.
- Scar management with lotion may be initiated.
- Manual desensitization exercises may be initiated as necessary. It is not uncommon for the patient to experience acute hypersensitivity along the incision site or in the surgical area in the early postoperation weeks. The desensitization exercises have proven quite effective in managing the sensitivity.
- Patient may begin light finger eating activities, use the hand as an assist in ADLs and use for bathing.

4 Weeks

- Patient can use hand for dressing ADLs with minimal resistance including pulling on socks and pants and reaching into back pocket.

S.F.M. Duncan and C.W. Flowers, *Therapy of the Hand and Upper Extremity: Rehabilitation Protocols*, DOI 10.1007/978-3-319-14412-2_21,
© Springer International Publishing Switzerland 2015

6–7 Weeks

• PROM to the elbow in extension may be initiated.

8–10 Weeks

• The patient may resume full use of the upper extremity in all daily activities.
• Restore strength in hypothenar and first dorsal interossei muscles.
• If the patient does have a fairly significant degree of persistent discomfort then the patient should gradually resume normal activity versus unrestricted activity.

Additional Comments

• It is important to carefully monitor the postoperative discomfort and to manage it fairly aggressively should it present itself. TENS has proven to be quite effective for quieting the discomfort. Often it is no longer needed after 3–4 weeks of treatment.
• It is important to be fairly aggressive with the scar management techniques as dense scar will often times form along the area of the incision site.
• As strengthening is initiated (particularly for the manual laborer) it is important that the strengthening be in a graded and progressive manner and that the patient not be overexercised or be expected to perform repetitive motions in the early postoperation weeks.

Discharge Criteria

• Independent in all dressing, eating, and hygiene activities. Begin use of hand in light housekeeping activities progressing to moderate.

Chapter 22
Radial Nerve Repair

0–3 Weeks

- Bulky compressive dressing.

3 Weeks

- The bulky dressing is removed and appropriate edema control applied.
- A wrist immobilization splint is applied in 30° of extension for continual wear.
- The splint is adjusted to decrease wrist extension by 10° each week until neutral is obtained by the sixth week.
- Active passive ROM exercises are initiated to all digits, no motion to wrist.
- Patient is able to perform light dressing activities and eating within the constraints of the splint.

6 Weeks

- The splint is discontinued.
- If radial nerve palsy is present, the splint should be worn to allow hand function and prevent wrist drop or radial nerve palsy splint may be fabricated.
- Active and passive ROM exercises are initiated to the wrist.
- Progressive strengthening is initiated.

S.F.M. Duncan and C.W. Flowers, *Therapy of the Hand and Upper Extremity: Rehabilitation Protocols*, DOI 10.1007/978-3-319-14412-2_22, © Springer International Publishing Switzerland 2015

- Patient is able to perform all dressing, eating, and hygiene activities.

***Note*: If repair is above the elbow, static elbow splint is fitted initially at 0° and flexion is increased to 30° per week until 90° is obtained by the sixth week.

Discharge Criteria

- Patient is independent in all activities of self-care and is beginning light-to-moderate household activities.

Chapter 23
Radial Tunnel Syndrome

0–6 Weeks

Splinting:

- A wrist immobilization splint is fitted to the patient in 45° of extension for continual wear for approximately 6 weeks.
- The patient is reevaluated by the physician for resolution of the clinical symptoms. The purpose of this splint is to quiet any potential irritation of the radial nerve from forceful extension and supination of the wrist and forearm.
- On occasion, an elbow splint may also be ordered.

Strengthening:

- Progressive strengthening is initiated to the upper extremity using putty, a hand helper, Theraband, and free weights once the symptoms have resolved.
- The patient is advised to:
  - Avoid a combination of forceful, repetitive wrist extension or supination unless necessary for job simulation.
  - Use two hands to lift when feasible.
  - Lift with the palms up when feasible (instead of palms down).
  - Use a tool with a longer lever arm when feasible.

S.F.M. Duncan and C.W. Flowers, *Therapy of the Hand and Upper Extremity: Rehabilitation Protocols*,
DOI 10.1007/978-3-319-14412-2_23,
© Springer International Publishing Switzerland 2015

○ Modify tools to decrease the amount of supination and wrist extension (i.e., pistol grip handles).

Additional Comments:

• When wrist immobilization splints are fitted, it is important that the proximal strap not be irritating in the area of the radial nerve.

Discharge Criteria

• More if soft tissue mobilization is part of MD order.
• Patient should be able to demonstrate proper body mechanics.

Chapter 24
Splinting for Nerve Palsies of the Upper Extremity

Splinting for Median Nerve

- Recommended splint: Web spacer.
- Purpose: Maintains thumb web space thereby preventing a first web space contracture. This is necessary due to paralysis of the thenar intrinsics.
- Precautions: Do not hyperextend the thumb MCP joint or stress the UCL of the MCP joint.
- Wearing time: The splint should be worn between exercises and at night.

Splinting for Ulnar Nerve

- Recommended splint: MCP extension block splint to the ring and small fingers or Wynn-Parry.
- Purpose: To prevent clawing of the ring and small fingers due to paralysis of the ulnar innervated intrinsics.
- Wearing time: Continuously until the MCP volar plates tighten, there is return of the intrinsics, or tendon transfers are performed.

Splinting of Combined Median and Ulnar Nerve

- Recommended splint: MCP extension block splint to index through small fingers or double Wynn-Parry.
- Purpose: To prevent clawing of the index through small fingers due to paralysis of the intrinsics.

S.F.M. Duncan and C.W. Flowers, *Therapy of the Hand and Upper Extremity: Rehabilitation Protocols*, DOI 10.1007/978-3-319-14412-2_24, © Springer International Publishing Switzerland 2015

- Wearing time: Continuously until the MCP volar plates tighten, there is return of the intrinsics, or tendon transfers are performed.

Splinting for Radial Nerve: Low

- Recommended splint: Wrist immobilization splint with or without dynamic.
- Purpose: To position the wrist in approximately 30° of extension to allow improved functional use of the hand and prevent wrist drop. Digits can be included to aid in MCP extension.
- Wearing time: The splint is worn until there is return of the radial nerve innervated muscles, or tendon transfers are performed.

Chapter 25
Ulnar and/or Median Nerve Repair

2 Weeks

- The bulky compressive dressing is removed.
- A dorsal blocking splint is fitted with the wrist in 30° of palmar flexion for continual wear.
- Ulnar nerve laceration only—the dorsal blocking splint includes the ring and small MCP joints in 30° of flexion to prevent clawing.
- Median nerve only—a web spacer splint is fitted to the thumb to wear at night to maintain the first web space.
- Combined median and ulnar nerve—the dorsal blocking splint includes the MCP joints of index through small; web spacer if fitted to wear at night.
- Active and passive ROM of digits and thumb each hour within DBS. Emphasize blocking exercises for long flexors. Scar massage and otoform 24 h following suture removal. FES may be used to enhance excursion of long flexors.
- Patient may begin light pickups within the constraints of the splint.

4–6 Weeks

- The splint is adjusted to increase wrist extension by 10 each week until neutral is obtained by the sixth week.
- Patient should be able to perform most dressing activities independently at this time.

S.F.M. Duncan and C.W. Flowers, *Therapy of the Hand and Upper Extremity: Rehabilitation Protocols*, DOI 10.1007/978-3-319-14412-2_25, © Springer International Publishing Switzerland 2015

6 Weeks

- The dorsal blocking splint is discontinued.
- The MCP extension block splint and/or web spacer is continued to prevent deformity.
- Active and passive ROM exercises are initiated to the wrist.
- Patient may bath without use of a splint.

7 Weeks

- Progressive strengthening is initiated.

Discharge Criteria

- Independent in all dressing, eating, and hygiene activities. Begin use of hand in light household activities progressing to moderate.

Part V
Elbow Sports Injuries

Chapter 26
Distal Biceps Repair

1–2 Weeks

- Minimize swelling and pain—TENS Unit/Ice prn
- Full forearm supination and pronation
- Elbow ROM from 30° of extension to 130° of flexion
- ROM Elbow as above 5–6 times per day (*ALL PASSIVE*)
- AROM Shoulder

3–6 Weeks

- Full elbow and forearm ROM by 6 weeks
- Week 3: *ACTIVE* Elbow extension limit changed to 20°. *PASSIVE* flexion may be increases to full flexion as tolerated
- Week 3: *ACTIVE* Wrist flexion extension, full-hand ROM, active supination/pronation
- Week 4: *ACTIVE* Elbow extension limit changed to 10°, begin Putty for grip strength, pulley ROM exercises (attend to extension limitation)
- Week 5: *ACTIVE* Elbow extension to full, begin supine scapular stabilizations (*no weight*), door ABCs or Circles with ball
- Week 6: *PASSIVE* Elbow extension to full as needed
- Week 6: Begin light tubing or 1-kg weights for elbow flexion/extension, forearm rotation and wrist flexion/extension, supine scapular stabilizations

S.F.M. Duncan and C.W. Flowers, *Therapy of the Hand and Upper Extremity: Rehabilitation Protocols*, DOI 10.1007/978-3-319-14412-2_26, © Springer International Publishing Switzerland 2015

- Week 6: Begin ball toss/trampoline toss, shoulder thera-band strengthening

3–6 Weeks

- Normalize elbow strength
- Begin strengthening exercises to wrist, forearm, and possibly shoulder, depending on sport and/or work requirements

  Full activity not recommended for 6 months

Chapter 27
Elbow Arthroscopy

1–2 Weeks

- Minimize swelling and pain—TENS Unit/Ice prn
- Full wrist and elbow ROM
- Retard muscle atrophy
- Begin putty grip strengthening
- Wrist flexor/extensor group stretching
- PROM/AAROM Elbow flexion/extension/pron/supin as tolerated—NO restrictions

3–4 Weeks

- Normalize joint arthrokinematics
- Improve muscular strength, power, and endurance
- Begin strengthening program (1 lb weight): flex/ext/neutral wrist curls, pronation/supination, broomstick rollup
- Begin biceps curls, triceps extensions, begin eccentrics at Week 4
- Begin rotator cuff strengthening program: IR/ER, deltoid, scapular stab

5–8 Weeks

- Prepare for return to functional activities
- Begin endurance and flexibility drills
- Return to sport-specific drills

S.F.M. Duncan and C.W. Flowers, *Therapy of the Hand and Upper Extremity: Rehabilitation Protocols*,
DOI 10.1007/978-3-319-14412-2_27,
© Springer International Publishing Switzerland 2015

Chapter 28
Elbow UCL Reconstruction

BRACE—Posterior splint at 90° Elbow flexion for Week 1, Transition to functional brace (30–100°) after Week 1.

1–3 Weeks

- Minimize pain at rest
- Restore Elbow ROM—Extension 30°, Flexion 130°
- Scapular and rotator cuff competency
- ROM: AROM within brace, increase brace ROM 10° flex and ext each week
- Begin hand, wrist, and shoulder AROM
- Scapular and rotator cuff exercises: active with some light resistive
- Begin light isometric/isotonic strengthening for wrist (and elbow as comfortable) (1 lb)

4–6 Weeks

- Full-elbow flexion, 0° extension, full supination/pronation
- 3/5 Wrist and elbow strength
- Scapular and rotator cuff strength 5/5
- Gradually progress elbow/wrist AROM/AAROM
- Progress scapular and rotator cuff strengthening with light resistance
- Increase elbow/wrist resistance to 1–3 lb

S.F.M. Duncan and C.W. Flowers, *Therapy of the Hand and Upper Extremity: Rehabilitation Protocols*, DOI 10.1007/978-3-319-14412-2_28, © Springer International Publishing Switzerland 2015

7–15 Weeks

- Full-elbow PROM
- 5/5 Strength—Rotator cuff, deltoid, wrist, elbow
- Gradually increase resistance (wrist/elbow) up to 10 lb
- Progress PROM to reach full ROM in all directions
- Begin manual resistance PNF patterns
- Begin light sport-specific activities at Week 11
- Begin light bilateral plyometric program

16+ Weeks

- Return to full activity
- Advanced strengthening, weight room activities
- Progress sport-specific activities
- For throwing athletes—begin interval throwing program at 5 months per MD

  *Begin competitive throwing between 7 and 9 months

- Begin single-arm eccentric strengthening

Chapter 29
Lateral Epicondyleplasty

0–2 Weeks

- Bulky compressive dressing is removed and patient is splinted in a long-arm splint with wrist in 20° extension, forearm neutral, and elbow at 90°.
- Patient removed the splint six times a day for elbow flexion and extension exercises.

3 Weeks

- Start wrist flexion/extension and supination/pronation.
- Interval splint.

4 Weeks

- Patient to begin gentle strengthening with putty.

5 Weeks

- D/C elbow splint.

6 Weeks

- D/C wrist splint.
- Forearm strengthening.

Discharge Criteria

- Independent in self-care activities beginning light lifting with minimal pain.

S.F.M. Duncan and C.W. Flowers, *Therapy of the Hand and Upper Extremity: Rehabilitation Protocols*, DOI 10.1007/978-3-319-14412-2_29, © Springer International Publishing Switzerland 2015

Chapter 30
Lateral Epicondylitis "Tennis Elbow" Nonoperative

4–8 Weeks

- A wrist immobilization splint is applied in 45° of extension for continual wear. The patient should then be reevaluated between 4 and 8 weeks. If the acute symptoms persist, continued immobilization may be necessary for an additional 4–6 weeks. Surgery may be necessary if the symptoms do not resolve from these conservative measures.
- A pneumatic arm band may be worn for comfort.
- Patient is educated on tendon protection techniques.

8–12 Weeks

- Begin gentle, progressive strengthening to the upper extremity using putty, hand helper, theraband, Nirschl exercises, and/or a formal work hardening program. The goal is to equally strengthen all muscle groups of the upper extremity.
- Patients may continue to use the pneumatic arm band during repetitive use of the upper extremity.
- Educate patient in proper body mechanics.
  - Lift with palms up whenever possible.
  - Use both upper extremities in such a way that it reduces the combined amount of forcible elbow extension, supination, and wrist extension.

S.F.M. Duncan and C.W. Flowers, *Therapy of the Hand and Upper Extremity: Rehabilitation Protocols*, DOI 10.1007/978-3-319-14412-2_30,
© Springer International Publishing Switzerland 2015

° Avoid forceful exertion with the wrists and elbows extended and the forearm pronated.

Progressive Protocol

0–2 Weeks

• Evaluate for pain level and trigger points make referral for ultrasound or iontophoresis as needed. Utilize soft tissue techniques with ice or heat as appropriate. Teach patient how to self-monitor symptoms and control the symptoms.
  ° Splint the wrist in 45° of extension to wear at all times.
  ° Begin forearm and wrist stretches during the day.
  ° Educate patients on activities that cause pain and develop independent joint protection techniques.
  ° Begin Nirschl exercise program one time per day with no weights.

2–4 Weeks

• Continue with stretches.
• Continue with modalities as needed but begin to wean off.
• Begin to decrease splint wear at home.
• If after a week pain level decreases or is maintained, initiate isometric exercises for HEP.
• Patient should be able to utilize joint protection and pain control techniques including ice and splinting to decrease problems.

4–6 Weeks

• With pain level decreasing or maintaining, add weight to Nirschl program.
• Modalities should be eliminated.
• Begin simulations as needed.
• Wean off splint for work.

6 Weeks

- Patient will be able to problem solve activities and modify the activity.
- Patient will be able to utilize independently home pain-control methods.
- Patient will be independent in a home-exercise program to maintain strength and eliminate further problems.

Discharge Criteria

- Patient will demonstrate correct tendon protection techniques in ADLs and self-manage symptoms.
- Average number of visits—6.

.

Chapter 31
Lateral Epicondylitis/ Extensor Carpi Radialis Brevis Release (Elbow)

1 Week

- Minimize swelling and pain—TENS Unit/Ice
- Full-wrist and finger ROM
- Begin shoulder shrugs
- AROM Shoulder, wrist, and hand (pain-free)

2 Weeks

- Full-elbow ROM
- Begin elbow ROM, gentle elbow/wrist stretches
- Begin stationary bicycle
- Begin aquatic therapy once incisions healed

3–6 Weeks

- Pain-free ADLs
- Begin UBE (min resistance)
- Begin Isometrics × 8 (box plus supination/pronation) (pain-free), hand squeezing exercises—putty/sponge
- Begin treadmill running progression program
- Begin elliptical trainer—light grip

S.F.M. Duncan and C.W. Flowers, *Therapy of the Hand and Upper Extremity: Rehabilitation Protocols*, DOI 10.1007/978-3-319-14412-2_31, © Springer International Publishing Switzerland 2015

7–10 Weeks

- Normalize elbow strength
- Begin PREs—flex/ext wrist curls, supination/pronation against resistance
- Pushup progression—wall to table to chair

11+ Weeks

- Return to full activities including sports
- Begin regular push-ups
- Begin weight-training

Chapter 32
Medial Epicondylitis Nonoperative

4–8 Weeks

- A wrist immobilization splint is applied in neutral to 10° volar flexion for 4–8 weeks for continual wear. If the symptoms persist, prolonged splinting may be necessary.
- Some patients not effectively managed with wrist splinting alone may require a static elbow splint, which secures the forearm in a neutral position with the elbow flexed at 90°.

8–12 Weeks

- As the symptoms become quiescent, progressive resistive exercise may be initiated. This may include use of the BTE, Nirschl exercise program, and theraband.

Discharge Criteria

- Patient will be able to perform ADLs without pain.
- Average number of visits—6.

S.F.M. Duncan and C.W. Flowers, *Therapy of the Hand and Upper Extremity: Rehabilitation Protocols*, DOI 10.1007/978-3-319-14412-2_32, © Springer International Publishing Switzerland 2015

Chapter 33
Medial and Lateral Epicondylectomy

3 Weeks

- The bulky compressive dressing is removed and appropriated edema control is initiated as needed.
- A static elbow splint is fitted with the elbow positioned in 90° of flexion to wear between exercise sessions and at night primarily for comfort and protection. The splint may be applied to either anterior or posterior for comfort. Patients which have no postoperative discomfort at this early point in time may not require an elbow splint.
- AROM exercises are initiated to the elbow, forearm, and wrist, 6–8 times a day for 10 min.
- Scar management techniques consisting of scar massage with lotion or the use of otoform or elastomer are initiated.
- TENS may be initiated if the patient is somewhat painful at the 3-week point.
- Patient is able to perform eating, dressing, and bathing activities.

6 Weeks

- PROM exercises are initiated to the elbow in conjunction with the AROM exercises. Exercises are increased to an hourly basis as needed.

S.F.M. Duncan and C.W. Flowers, *Therapy of the Hand and Upper Extremity: Rehabilitation Protocols*, DOI 10.1007/978-3-319-14412-2_33, © Springer International Publishing Switzerland 2015

- Gentle strengthening may be initiated using putty and progressing to a hand helper, theraband, the BTE work simulator and the Nirschl exercise program. It is important to strengthen all muscle groups equally and to very gradually add graded resistance to the upper extremity. Patients who are returning to a work environment in which some degree or repetitive activity is performed should generally be placed on a return-to-work program at this time to ensure ability for return by 14–16 weeks.
- Patient is able to complete all dressing, hygiene, and light housekeeping and light work activities independently.

Discharge Criteria

- Patient will be independent in all activities except for lifting over 5 lb and push–pull activities with resistance.
- Average number of visits—10.

Chapter 34
Triceps Reconstruction

BRACE—Posterior splint at 90° Elbow flexion for Week 1, Transition to functional brace (30–100°) after Week 1

1–3 Weeks

- Minimize pain at rest
- Restore Elbow ROM—Extension 30°, Flexion 90°
- Scapular and rotator cuff competency
- ROM: AROM within brace, increase brace ROM 10° flex and ext each week
- Begin hand, wrist, and shoulder AROM
- Scapular and rotator cuff exercises: Active with some light resistive
- Scapular and rotator cuff exercises: Active with some light resistive
- Begin light isometric/isotonic strengthening for wrist (and elbow as comfortable) (1 lb)

4–6 Weeks

- Full-elbow flexion, 0° extension, full supination/pronation
- 3/5 Wrist and elbow strength
- Scapular and rotator cuff strength 5/5
- Gradually progress elbow/wrist AROM/AAROM
- Progress scapular and rotator cuff strengthening with light resistance
- Increase elbow/wrist resistance to 1–3 lb

S.F.M. Duncan and C.W. Flowers, *Therapy of the Hand and Upper Extremity: Rehabilitation Protocols*, DOI 10.1007/978-3-319-14412-2_34,
© Springer International Publishing Switzerland 2015

7–15 Weeks

- Full-elbow PROM
- 5/5 Strength—Rotator cuff, deltoid, wrist, elbow
- Gradually increase resistance (wrist/elbow) up to 10 lb
- Progress PROM to reach full ROM in all directions
- Begin manual resistance PNF patterns
- Begin light sport-specific activities at Week 11
- Begin light bilateral plyometric program

16 ± Weeks

- Return to full activity
- Advanced strengthening, weight room activities
- Progress sport-specific activities
- For throwing athletes—begin interval throwing program at 5 months per MD

   *   Begin competitive throwing between 7 and 9 months

- Begin single-arm eccentric strengthening

Part VI
Elbow Trauma

Chapter 35
Above or Below the Elbow Amputation

0–3 Weeks

- Initiate wound care: Dressings, debridement PRN.
- Decrease swelling. Apply light compressive dressings, ace wraps or coban.
- Minimize pain at rest.
- Allow wound to heal.
- Initiate active or active assistance ROM exercises to all remaining bilateral upper extremity joints. Perform the exercises with both limbs. Use a mirror to provide visual feedback and to help with phantom limb pain.
- TENS may be used PRN for pain.

3–8 Weeks

- Begin scar desensitization.
- Apply stump shrinker.
- Progressive strengthening may be initiated as appropriate for the level of amputation.
- Patient may begin ADLs as tolerated once the wound has closed.

***Appointment with prosthetist as soon as wound healed and edema controlled.
***Begin targeted therapies depending on type of prosthesis at 1 month.

S.F.M. Duncan and C.W. Flowers, *Therapy of the Hand and Upper Extremity: Rehabilitation Protocols*, DOI 10.1007/978-3-319-14412-2_35, © Springer International Publishing Switzerland 2015

Chapter 36
Distal Humerus Fracture ORIF

0–3 Weeks

- Apply edema control as needed.
- Apply long-arm splint, elbow in 90° of flexion, forearm in neutral, and wrist in 0–15° of extension.
- Initiate shoulder and digit ROM.

10 Days–3 Weeks

- Begin gentle active ROM including, elbow, forearm, and wrist.
- Hand strengthening including putty progressing to putty may be initiated.

4–6 Weeks

- Active assistive and passive motion may begin.

6–8 Weeks

- Begin progressive strengthening.

Discharge Criteria

- Independent in all self-care beginning light household activities.
- Average number of visits—15.

S.F.M. Duncan and C.W. Flowers, *Therapy of the Hand and Upper Extremity: Rehabilitation Protocols*, DOI 10.1007/978-3-319-14412-2_36, © Springer International Publishing Switzerland 2015

Chapter 37
Elbow Resection Arthroplasty

1 Week

- Patient begins CPM, and active and passive ROM to the elbow including supination and pronation.
- Patient is fitted with a static elbow splint to wear between exercises for comfort.
  - *Note*: Exercises during the initial 6 weeks of therapy should be performed at the patient's side. This may be reduced to 4 weeks in the patient with a stable, pain-free arc of motion.

3–4 Weeks

- Depending on the patient's comfort level and stability of the elbow, light functional activities may be initiated.
- The splint may be discontinued at this time.

6 Weeks

- Exercises and normal activities may be performed with the arm away from the patient's side.

S.F.M. Duncan and C.W. Flowers, *Therapy of the Hand and Upper Extremity: Rehabilitation Protocols*, DOI 10.1007/978-3-319-14412-2_37, © Springer International Publishing Switzerland 2015

Chapter 38
Radial Head Fractures, Olecranon Fractures, and Elbow Dislocation

Radial Head Fracture (Type I, II, and III with Excision of the Head)

- 0–10 Days
  - Splint with posterior elbow splint or sling.
  - Begin shoulder, digit, and wrist ROM.
- 5–10 Days
  - Begin AROM elbow and forearm.
  - Begin putty strengthening.
- 3–4 Weeks
  - Begin PROM and dynamic or static extension splinting.
- 4–6 Weeks
  - Begin progressive strengthening.

Radial Head Fracture (Type IV)

- 0–5 Days
  - Begin AROM in hinged splint.
  - Initiated shoulder, wrist, and hand ROM.

S.F.M. Duncan and C.W. Flowers, *Therapy of the Hand and Upper Extremity: Rehabilitation Protocols*, DOI 10.1007/978-3-319-14412-2_38, © Springer International Publishing Switzerland 2015

- 4 Weeks
  - Discontinued elbow splinting.
- 6–8 Weeks
  - Begin progressive strengthening program.

Discharge Criteria

- Independent in all self-care activities.

Part VII
Wrist Bone Injuries

Chapter 39
Wrist Arthrodesis

0–3 Days

- Begin digit ROM & digit edema control.

10–14 Days

- Remove surgical dressing, replace with light compressive dressing, along with bivalve wrist splint or the patient may be placed in a long-arm cast.
- Continue with digit AROM and PROM. Maximize excursion of the extensor tendons to prevent extrinsic extensor tightness.
- Begin scar management of suture area.
- Utilize TENS on the high rate as needed for postoperative pain, placement is along the radial nerve distribution.
- Also include shoulder, elbow, and forearm motion.
- If extensor lag develops a static night extension splint can be fabricated.
- If extrinsic extensor tightness develops dynamic flexion, splinting or FES (functional electric stimulation) may be utilized.

3 Weeks

- Upper arm strengthening can begin utilizing strap weights.

S.F.M. Duncan and C.W. Flowers, *Therapy of the Hand and Upper Extremity: Rehabilitation Protocols*,
DOI 10.1007/978-3-319-14412-2_39,
© Springer International Publishing Switzerland 2015

6 Weeks

- Putty strengthening can be initiated.

8–10 Weeks

- Splint may be discontinued with MD approval.

Discharge Criteria

- Independent self-care with the exception of toileting and fastening bra behind back.

Chapter 40
Wrist Arthroplasty

2–4 Weeks

- Remove surgical dressing, replace with light compressive dressing, along with bivalve wrist splint or short-arm cast.
- Begin shoulder, elbow, and finger motion.

4–6 Weeks

- Edema control.
- Begin scar management of suture area.
- AROM and PROM to wrist, hand, and fingers.
- Fit wrist splint at 15° extension worn at night and between exercises.
- Initiate dynamic splinting to increase PROM.
- Electrical stimulation PRN.

6 Weeks

- Focus on Full PROM.
- Begin ADL training.
- Discontinue wrist splint.

8 Weeks

- Gentle progressive strengthening of wrist, hand, and fingers.
- Putty strengthening exercises.

S.F.M. Duncan and C.W. Flowers, *Therapy of the Hand and Upper Extremity: Rehabilitation Protocols*, DOI 10.1007/978-3-319-14412-2_40, © Springer International Publishing Switzerland 2015

12 Weeks

- Simulate daily activities and progress to full activity

Discharge Criteria

- Independent self-care with the exception of toileting and fastening bra behind back.

Chapter 41
Bennett Fracture

6 Weeks

- The short-arm thumb spica cast (SATS) is removed assuming the fracture is clinically healed.
- Active and passive ROM exercises are initiated to the thumb approximately 10 min each hour.
- A thumb spica splint is fitted to wear between exercise session and at night.

8 Weeks

- Assuming the fracture is healed, the splint may be discontinued.
- Taping and/or dynamic flexion splinting may be initiated as necessary to increase passive ROM.
- Gentle strengthening may be initiated with putty and/or a hand exerciser.

10 Weeks

- Patients may generally return to normal activities.

S.F.M. Duncan and C.W. Flowers, *Therapy of the Hand and Upper Extremity: Rehabilitation Protocols*, DOI 10.1007/978-3-319-14412-2_41, © Springer International Publishing Switzerland 2015

Chapter 42
Chronic Osteoarthritis or Rheumatoid Arthritis Nonoperative

Initial Evaluation

- ROM measurements
- Grip strength
- Edema measurements
- Pain assessment
- ADL assessment

Intervention

- Patient education on joint protection and energy conservation
- Review adaptive equipment
- Home-exercise program as indicated

  - AROM
  - PROM
  - Strengthening

- Protective splinting PRN
- Use of thermal modalities

  - Moist heat
  - Paraffin
  - Ice

- Referral to community resources

S.F.M. Duncan and C.W. Flowers, *Therapy of the Hand and Upper Extremity: Rehabilitation Protocols*, DOI 10.1007/978-3-319-14412-2_42, © Springer International Publishing Switzerland 2015

***Note*: Patient is seen one time for initial evaluation and home program of patient education, exercise, splinting, and thermal modalities as indicated by the evaluation. Patient will return for follow up to determine effectiveness of home program as needed.

Discharge Criteria

- Demonstrated self-management skills for pain, edema, joint protection, and energy conservation.

Chapter 43
CMC Resection or Implant Arthroplasty

Immediately

1. Edema control:

   - The patient is instructed in edema control measures to minimize and reduce swelling. This should include light compression sleeves (coban) and decongestive massage. Emphasis should also be placed on elevation of the involved arm above the level of the heart when walking, sitting, or sleeping if possible. The use of a sling should be discouraged to prevent shoulder problems.

2. AROM of the uninvolved joints:

   - Active range of motion exercises for the uninvolved joints including the shoulder, elbow, fingers, and thumb IP should be encouraged.

4 Weeks

The thumb spica cast and surgical dressing are removed. In addition the sutures and percutaneous pins are removed.

1. Splint:
   A forearm-based orthoplast thumb spica with the IP free is fabricated to be worn fulltime except for exercises and bathing.

S.F.M. Duncan and C.W. Flowers, *Therapy of the Hand and Upper Extremity: Rehabilitation Protocols*, DOI 10.1007/978-3-319-14412-2_43,
© Springer International Publishing Switzerland 2015

2. Exercises:

At 4 weeks, active range of motion exercises can be initiated for the thumb. The exercises should be done 3–4 times a day, 10–15 repetitions, in a slow and pain-free manner. Specific emphasis should be placed on the following:

- Thumb MP and IP flexion, with caution not to hyperextend past neutral
- Gentle radial and palmar abduction (avoid excessive adduction)
- Opposition without stressing the thumb; gradually progress towards the small digit
- Wrist flexion and extension

3. Scar Management:

Friction massage can be initiated to be healed incision to help decrease the risk of adhesion. For night-time use, a silicone gel pad is useful to prevent scar tissue formation and provide pressure over the area. In addition, the patient should use vitamin E lotion or cocoa butter to help soften and desensitize the incision. It may also be necessary to provide further sensory reeducation should the incision be hypersensitive in nature.

6 Weeks

- Continue the exercise program as outlined at 4 weeks. The patient may now, however, begin gentle isometric strengthening exercises including thenar-cone muscle setting isometric exercises. Isometric strengthening should concentrate on all major muscle groups for the thumb and always be PAIN-FREE.
- Light functional activities can be added to the program to improve functional use of the hand and thumb. Caution should be taken to avoid any repetitive or heavy use of the involved hand at this time.
- Continue use of the thumb splint between exercises and functional activities. Upon the surgeon's discretion, the patient may now begin gradual weaning from the splint as tolerated.

8 Weeks

- Gentle isotonic grip and pinch strengthening can be initiated using soft theraputty.
- A program of progressive strengthening exercises and functional activities should be outlined until week 12–14.

Treatment Goal

Obtaining a stable, mobile, functional, and pain-free thumb.

Chapter 44
CMC Fracture or Dislocation

0–2 Weeks

- Keep bulky compressive dressing intact.

2 Weeks

- The bulky dressing is removed.
- Appropriate edema control is applied.
- A wrist immobilization splint is fitted for continual wear.
- Active and gentle passive ROM exercises are initiated to the digits 10 min/h.
- FES may be added to facilitate tendon excursion of hand flexors or extensors.

3–4 Weeks

- Assuming the fracture/dislocation is clinically stable and healing: AROM exercises are initiated to the wrist and forearm 6 times/day.
- Dynamic splinting may be initiated to the digits PRN.
- Wrist splint is worn between exercises and at night.

6 Weeks

- PROM exercises are initiated to the wrist and forearm.

S.F.M. Duncan and C.W. Flowers, *Therapy of the Hand and Upper Extremity: Rehabilitation Protocols*, DOI 10.1007/978-3-319-14412-2_44, © Springer International Publishing Switzerland 2015

- Dynamic splinting or wrist CPM may be used PRN to increase wrist ROM.

8 Weeks

- Gentle, progressive strengthening is initiated.

Chapter 45
Darrach Procedure

0–3 Weeks

- The patient remains in a bulky compressive dressing with the elbow flexed at 90° and the forearm supinated.
- If dressing soiled or uncomfortable, ok to remove the bulky dressing at 2 weeks postoperation and fit the patient with a long arm splint in the same position.
- Initiate digit ROM—no forearm rotation.

3 Weeks

- Wrist immobilization splint fitted in 15° of extension to wear between exercise sessions and at night for comfort.
- Active ROM and passive ROM exercises to the wrist and forearm on an hourly basis.
- As passive ROM exercises are performed to the forearm it is important to be sure to do the PROM proximal to the wrist and not distally by turning the hand.
- Patient may begin light eating, bathing, and dressing activities at this time.

  ◦ *Note*: The patient may have some degree of discomfort along the area of the distal ulna as forearm rotation is attempted. This discomfort generally diminishes by 6 weeks postoperation.
  ◦ *Note*: If the Darrach is performed along with multiple procedures in a rheumatoid, active ROM exercises may

S.F.M. Duncan and C.W. Flowers, *Therapy of the Hand and Upper Extremity: Rehabilitation Protocols*,
DOI 10.1007/978-3-319-14412-2_45,
© Springer International Publishing Switzerland 2015

be when the bulky dressing is initially taken down (3–5 days postoperation). Generally, AROM exercises are initiated at this early time frame. If the surgical area for the Darrach is painful, exercises may need to be minimized in the initial weeks postoperatively.

○ *Note*: Some patients are noted to have a slight dorsal subluxation of the distal ulna and find it much more comfortable to have a distal ulna strap applied approximately two inches proximal to the distal ulna to assist with keeping the distal ulna in an anatomic position. If the patient is noted to have persistent subluxation, there may be a moderate amount of pain which would then need to be reevaluated by the physician.

6 Weeks

The wrist immobilization splint may be discontinued so long as the patient is non-painful.

Gentle strengthening exercises may be initiated.

Discharge Criteria

• Patient should be independent with writing, eating, cutting food, hygiene, and dressing.

Chapter 46
Distal Radius Fracture: External Fixation

0–4 Weeks

- A long arm splint is applied for continual wear.
- Active and passive ROM exercises are initiated to the digits 15 min/h and to the elbow and shoulder as needed.
- Appropriated edema control is applied.
- Pin care is performed daily.
- Forearm supination/pronation is initiated with M.D. clearance.

4–6 Weeks (Fracture Is Clinically Stable)

- External fixation is removed.
- A wrist immobilization splint is fitted to wear between exercises and at night.
- Active ROM exercises are initiated to the wrist and forearm 8 times a day.
- Grip strengthening is initiated with putty and/or hand helper.

6–8 Weeks (Fracture Is Clinically Healed)

- Passive ROM exercises are initiated to the wrist and forearm 8 times a day.
- Wrist and upper strengthening is initiated.
- Begin light ADLs with interval splinting.

S.F.M. Duncan and C.W. Flowers, *Therapy of the Hand and Upper Extremity: Rehabilitation Protocols*, DOI 10.1007/978-3-319-14412-2_46, © Springer International Publishing Switzerland 2015

8–10 Weeks

- The splint is discontinued.
- Light normal use is allowed.

12 Weeks

- Unrestricted use is allowed.

Discharge Criteria

- Independent all self-care except for fastening bra behind back and reaching into pocket.

Chapter 47
Distal Radius Fracture Nonoperative

0–4 Weeks

- A short arm cast, or long arm cast is applied.
- Active and passive range of motion exercises are initiated to the digits, elbow, and shoulder, as needed (this can include finger taping). Once patient is put in a short arm cast, forearm rotation may begin.
- Edema control is applied to the digits PRN.

  ○ Note: Monitor for increased levels of edema and pain which may result in dystrophy.

4–6 Weeks

- Cast is removed when sufficient healing is present.
- Wrist immobilization splint is applied to wear between exercises and at night.
- Active ROM exercises are initiated to the wrist and forearm 8 times a day.
- FES for thumb, digits, wrist, and forearm.
- Edema control PRN.
- Patient may begin light ADLs with splint on.

6–8 Weeks

- Passive ROM exercises are initiated to the wrist and forearm 8 times a day.

S.F.M. Duncan and C.W. Flowers, *Therapy of the Hand and Upper Extremity: Rehabilitation Protocols*,
DOI 10.1007/978-3-319-14412-2_47,
© Springer International Publishing Switzerland 2015

- Grip strengthening with putty and/or hand helper is initiated.
- Dynamic splinting wrist and/or forearm 4–6 times a day.
- Begin light ADLs without splint.

8–10 Weeks

- The splint is discontinued.
- Wrist strengthening is initiated.
- Light normal use is resumed.

12 Weeks

- Full normal use is resumed.

Discharge Criteria

- Independent self-care with difficulty with fastening bra behind back and reaching into back pocket.

Chapter 48
Distal Radius Fracture ORIF

0–4 Weeks

- A short arm cast, or long arm cast is applied.
- Active and passive range of motion exercises are initiated to the digits, elbow, and shoulder, as needed. Once patient is put in a short arm cast, forearm rotation may begin.
- Begin intrinsic muscle strengthening and tendon gliding exercises to the hand/digits.
- Edema control is applied to the digits PRN.

  ○ *Note*: Monitor for increased levels of edema and pain which may result in dystrophy.

4–6 Weeks

- Cast is removed when sufficient healing is present.
- Wrist immobilization splint is applied to wear between exercises and at night.
- Passive and Active Assist ROM exercises are initiated to the wrist and forearm 8 times a day.
- FES for thumb, digits, wrist, and forearm.
- Edema control PRN.

6–8 Weeks

- Begin Active ROM.
- Dynamic splinting wrist and/or forearm 4–6 times a day.
- Patient may begin light ADLs with splint on.

S.F.M. Duncan and C.W. Flowers, *Therapy of the Hand and Upper Extremity: Rehabilitation Protocols*,
DOI 10.1007/978-3-319-14412-2_48,
© Springer International Publishing Switzerland 2015

8–10 Weeks

- Patient may begin ADLs without splint.
- Grip strengthening with putty and/or hand helper is initiated.

10–12 Weeks

- Wrist strengthening is initiated.
- Light normal use is resumed.

12 Weeks

- Full normal use is resumed.

Discharge Criteria

- Independent self-care with difficulty with fastening bra behind back and reaching into back pocket.

Chapter 49
Four-Corner Fusion

2–4 Weeks

- Remove stitches and exchange splint (we prefer thumb spica).
- PROM and AROM to fingers.

4–8 Weeks

- Slow and gentle PROM and AROM to wrist.
- Edema control.
- Scar desensitization.
- Splint to be used around the clock except at night or during bathing or exercises.

8–16 Weeks

- Discontinue splint.
- Progress AROM.
- Begin strengthening once fusion indicated by MD.

Discharge Criteria

- Patient will be independent in dressing, hygiene, and eating progressing to light household activities.

S.F.M. Duncan and C.W. Flowers, *Therapy of the Hand and Upper Extremity: Rehabilitation Protocols*, DOI 10.1007/978-3-319-14412-2_49, © Springer International Publishing Switzerland 2015

Chapter 50
Proximal Row Carpectomy

10 Days

- The bulky compressive dressing is removed and the patient is fitted with a short arm cast.
- Active and passive ROM exercises are initiated to the digits and to the thumb.

4 Weeks

- Edema control may be initiated as necessary.
- Scar management may be initiated with scar massage and lotion or the use of otoform.
- Active, assistive, and gentle passive ROM exercises may be initiated to the wrist, thumb, and fingers.
- A wrist immobilization splint is fitted to wear between exercise sessions and at night. The primary purpose of the wrist splint is for comfort and support.
- The patient should be gradually weaned out of the wrist splint by 8 weeks.

8 Weeks

- Progressive strengthening may be initiated with a hand helper or putty and gentle weighted resistance.
- Discontinue splinting if possible.

S.F.M. Duncan and C.W. Flowers, *Therapy of the Hand and Upper Extremity: Rehabilitation Protocols*,
DOI 10.1007/978-3-319-14412-2_50,
© Springer International Publishing Switzerland 2015

Discharge Criteria

- Patient will be independent in dressing, hygiene, and eating progressing to light household activities.

Chapter 51
Scaphoid Fracture Nonoperative

12–20 Weeks

- *Cast immobilization*:
    - *Proximal pole*: immobilization in LATSC for approximately 16–20 weeks.
    - *Central portion*: immobilization in LATSC for approximately 3 months.
    - *Distal portion*: immobilization in LATSC for approximately 6–8 weeks.

Following Immobilization

- AROM exercises are initiated to the forearm, wrist, and thumb 6–8 times a day following the prolonged immobilization.
- A wrist and thumb static splint is fitted with the wrist in neutral to be worn between exercise sessions and at night.
- PROM exercises, dynamic wrist splinting, and strengthening exercises may be initiated once the fracture is radiographically or clinically healed as determined by the surgeon.

S.F.M. Duncan and C.W. Flowers, *Therapy of the Hand and Upper Extremity: Rehabilitation Protocols*, DOI 10.1007/978-3-319-14412-2_51, © Springer International Publishing Switzerland 2015

Chapter 52
Scaphoid Fracture ORIF

0–2 Weeks

- Edema control. Limb elevation, compressive wrap over thumb spica splint.
- Begin shoulder, elbow, and finger ROM.

2–6 Weeks

- Exchange to removable thumb spica splint.
- Continue edema control.
- Gentle PROM of wrist advancing as tolerated to gentle AROM.
- Scar desensitization.
- Splint continuously on except bathing and therapy sessions.

6–12 Weeks

- Discontinue splint.
- Await MD clearance of union.
- Advance AROM of wrist.
- Begin strengthening once union.

S.F.M. Duncan and C.W. Flowers, *Therapy of the Hand and Upper Extremity: Rehabilitation Protocols*, DOI 10.1007/978-3-319-14412-2_52, © Springer International Publishing Switzerland 2015

Chapter 53
Sauve-Kapanji Lowenstein Procedure

2 Weeks

- The bulky compressive dressing is removed and edema control is applied as needed.
- A long arm splint is applied and worn for approximately 6 more weeks.
- Active and passive ROM exercises are initiated to the digits as well as to the shoulder.

8 Weeks

- The long arm splint is discontinued.
- Active and active assistive ROM exercises are initiated to the wrist and forearm on an hourly basis.
- PROM exercises are initiated when the fusion is clinically and/or radiographically healed.
- Dynamic splinting to the wrist and forearm may be initiated assuming the patient's pain and discomfort are at a minimum.
- Patient may use extremity for bathing and assist in dressing.

***Note**: If the free end of the ulna appears to float, a strap around the forearm may provide additional support.

S.F.M. Duncan and C.W. Flowers, *Therapy of the Hand and Upper Extremity: Rehabilitation Protocols*,
DOI 10.1007/978-3-319-14412-2_53,
© Springer International Publishing Switzerland 2015

Discharge Criteria

- Patient is independent in all dressing except for fastening bra behind the back and reaching into back pocket, bathing, and hygiene.

Part VIII
Wrist Ligament/Soft Tissue Injuries

Chapter 54
CMC Soft Tissue Reconstruction

0–6 Weeks

- Thumb spica cast.
  - Active and passive ROM exercises are initiated to the digits PRN.
- Thumb spica splint.
  - Active and passive ROM exercises are initiated to the digits PRN.
  - Edema control as needed.
  - Instruct in pin care.
  - Begin AROM of IP and MCP with CMC joint stabilized.
  - No activities are permitted with the thumb at this time.

4–6 Weeks

- The cast is removed.
- A thumb spica splint is fitted to wear between exercises and at night.
- Appropriate edema control methods are implemented; scar massage and otoform are initiated.
- Active and passive ROM exercises are initiated to the thumb and wrist 15 min/h, including thumb taping.
- Patient may begin light pick up activities including finger eating and use as assist in bathing.

S.F.M. Duncan and C.W. Flowers, *Therapy of the Hand and Upper Extremity: Rehabilitation Protocols*,
DOI 10.1007/978-3-319-14412-2_54,
© Springer International Publishing Switzerland 2015

7 Weeks

- Dynamic thumb flexion splinting may be initiated PRN with stabilization of the CMC joint.
  - The splint may be reduced to hand based.
  - Patient may begin light utensil use.

8 Weeks

- The splint is continued PRN for protection or discontinued if pain is minimal.
- Gentle, progressive strengthening is initiated if patient is pain free.
- Patient may begin progressing resistive pinch activities.

Discharge Criteria

- Patient is able to write with some discomfort, pull up pants, initiate squeezing a bottle, and turn the key in the ignition.
- Average number of visits—8.

***Additional Comments*: Some patients may develop hypersensitivity of the suture and pin sites, and thus a desensitization program is appropriate to begin.

Chapter 55
Ganglionectomy

0–1 Week

- Bulky compressive dressing.

1 Week

- The bulky compressive dressing is removed.
- Edema control is initiated.
- Once sutures are removed, scar management is initiated.
- Putty strengthening is initiated PRN.
- Wrist and/or digit ROM is initiated as needed.

Discharge Criteria

- Independent in all dressing activities.
- Independent with cutting food with a knife and fork.
- Able to lift a 16 oz container and pour fluid from it.
- Independent in all bathing and grooming activities.

S.F.M. Duncan and C.W. Flowers, *Therapy of the Hand and Upper Extremity: Rehabilitation Protocols*,
DOI 10.1007/978-3-319-14412-2_55,
© Springer International Publishing Switzerland 2015

Chapter 56
Triangular Fibrocartilage Complex Repair (TFCC)

2 Weeks

- Remove bulky compressive long arm dressing.
- Fit the patient with either a long arm cast or long arm splint with the forearm supinated and the elbow flexed to 90° for continual wear.

6 Weeks

- The patient is fitted with either a short arm cast or a wrist immobilization splint.
- AROM exercises may be initiated to the elbow and forearm 10 min each hour.
- Patient should be independent utilizing op hand as assist in ADLs with splint on.

12 Weeks

- Active, active assistive, and gentle passive ROM exercises are initiated to the wrist, forearm, and elbow.
- A wrist immobilization splint is worn between exercise sessions and at night.
- Patient should be independent in bathing, dressing, and eating without splint.

  ***Note*: The splint may be discontinued when the patient is relatively pain free along the ulnar side of wrist.

S.F.M. Duncan and C.W. Flowers, *Therapy of the Hand and Upper Extremity: Rehabilitation Protocols*, DOI 10.1007/978-3-319-14412-2_56, © Springer International Publishing Switzerland 2015

12–14 Weeks

- Progressive strengthening may be initiated.

Discharge Criteria

- Patient will be independent in all dressing, hygiene, and self-care activities.
- Patient will be independent in lifting a 32 fluid container.
- Patient will be independent and pain free opening doors.

Chapter 57
Wrist Sprain/Contusion

1–2 Weeks

- A wrist immobilization splint is fitted to wear between exercises and at night.
- Wrist ROM exercises are initiated four times a day for 15 min sessions.
- Pain control as needed.
- Independent finger eating.

2–3 Weeks

- Patient is weaned from splint wear as tolerated.
- Light normal use is encouraged. Patient should be able to bathe with involved hand and use hand as assist in dressing.
- ROM exercises are continued.
- Strengthening is initiated to hand and upper extremity with putty, hand helper, and Nirschl program as appropriate.

3–4 Weeks

- The splint is discontinued.
- Normal use of the hand is resumed.
- Referral to Work Hardening if patient unable to return to work.

S.F.M. Duncan and C.W. Flowers, *Therapy of the Hand and Upper Extremity: Rehabilitation Protocols*,
DOI 10.1007/978-3-319-14412-2_57,
© Springer International Publishing Switzerland 2015

Discharge Criteria

- Independent all dressing, eating, hygiene, and self-care.
- Able to lift 32 oz container of fluid and pull open door and push door with difficulty.

Part IX
Wrist: Nerve Compression

Chapter 58
Carpal Tunnel Release Endoscopic

0–2 Weeks

- Edema control PRN.
- Active/passive ROM of digits.
- Scar massage.
- Patient able to use hand for bathing once sutures are removed.

2–4 Weeks

- Active/passive ROM of wrist and putty strengthening.
- Progress activities of daily living from light to normal.
- Scar management and desensitization.
- Patient education regarding proper body mechanics: maintain the wrist in neutral, avoid sustained grip/pinch for extended periods of time.

Discharge Criteria

- Independent in all self-care and dressing activities.

S.F.M. Duncan and C.W. Flowers, *Therapy of the Hand and Upper Extremity: Rehabilitation Protocols*, DOI 10.1007/978-3-319-14412-2_58, © Springer International Publishing Switzerland 2015

Chapter 59
Carpal Tunnel Release (Open)

0–6 Weeks

- Promote healing of wound
- Control pain and inflammation
- Restore full PROM/AROM in wrist and digits

1–3 Weeks

- Week 2—Begin tendon gliding program, thumb flexion/extension, and opposition AROM exercises, gentle wrist flexion and extension AROM, as well as elbow and shoulder AROM exercises 3–5 times/day
- Median nerve gliding exercises 3–5 times/day

4–6 Weeks

- Add gentle composite hand/wrist extension
- Begin light exercises against resistance: squeezing ball/foam, three-point and lateral pinch with theraputty, power web, and hand gripping exercises
- Begin gentle activities of daily living

7–12 Weeks

- Goals:
  - Restore full ROM in wrist/hand
  - Progress strength

S.F.M. Duncan and C.W. Flowers, *Therapy of the Hand and Upper Extremity: Rehabilitation Protocols*,
DOI 10.1007/978-3-319-14412-2_59,
© Springer International Publishing Switzerland 2015

- Prepare for return to work at 8 weeks for sedentary jobs, 10–12 for heavier jobs, or per MD clearance
- Exercises (7–8 Weeks):
  - Begin wrist curls with graded weight (flex/ext/sup/pron/radial and ulnar deviation)
  - Begin bicep curls and shoulder strengthening exercises if weak/atrophy
- Exercises (9–12 Weeks):
  - Return to daily functional activities, full clearance by MD

Chapter 60
Carpal Tunnel Nonoperative

0–4 Weeks

- Wrist immobilization splint in 15° of extension for continual wear.
- The patient is then reevaluated by the physician.
- A conservative exercise program consisting of isolated tendon blocking and AROM to the wrist.
- Modalities are utilized as indicated.
- If conservative management resolves symptoms, then gradual, progressive strengthening is initiated, and the splint wear is gradually decreased.
- Educate on nerve protection techniques and movement precautions, including: maintain the wrist in neutral position, avoid sustained pinch/grip, particularly pinching with the wrist in flexion, and avoid repetitive overuse of the wrist in activity.
- All ADLs are performed with splint on except for bathing.

Discharge Criteria

- Patient is able to demonstrate use of splint in all activities.
- Patient is able to demonstrate use of proper positioning in ADLs.

S.F.M. Duncan and C.W. Flowers, *Therapy of the Hand and Upper Extremity: Rehabilitation Protocols*, DOI 10.1007/978-3-319-14412-2_60, © Springer International Publishing Switzerland 2015

Part X
Wrist Tendon Injuries

Chapter 61
Camitz Transfer PL to APB Transfer

3 Weeks

- Remove bulky compression dressing.
- Initiate appropriate edema control measures PRN.
- Apply wrist and thumb static splint with the thumb positioned in wide palmar abduction and the wrist in 0° flexion for continual wear. The IP joint on the thumb is left free in the splint.
- Begin ROM of the forearm, elbow, and digits.
- Begin scar management once sutures are removed.
- No use of hand without splint.

4 Weeks

- Active and gentle passive ROM exercises are initiated to the thumb and wrist for 10 min sessions each hour.
- The splint is continued between exercises and at night.
- Patient may begin light feeding activities and use as assist in dressing.

6 Weeks

- The splint is discontinued altogether.
- Progressive strengthening may be initiated beginning with a nerf ball and soft putty.
- Patient may use hand for dressing, eating, and light hygiene.

S.F.M. Duncan and C.W. Flowers, *Therapy of the Hand and Upper Extremity: Rehabilitation Protocols*, DOI 10.1007/978-3-319-14412-2_61, © Springer International Publishing Switzerland 2015

Discharge Criteria

- Patient will be independent in dressing, hygiene, and eating progressing to light household activities.

Chapter 62
DeQuervain's Tenosynovitis Nonoperative

0–6 Weeks

- A wrist and thumb static splint with the IP joint free is fitted for continual wear for a period of 6 weeks. The splint is fabricated in the following:

  - Wrist: 15 of extension
  - Thumb CMC: 40 palmar abduction
  - Thumb MP: 10 of flexion
  - Thumb IP: Do not immobilize

6 Weeks

- Reevaluation by the surgeon.
- If symptoms are quiescent or have reduced significantly then nonoperative management is continued. If the symptoms are persisting at the same level of discomfort, surgical intervention may be considered or continuation of the nonoperative management splinting program.

**Patient education, it is important to advise the patient on the following:

- Avoid thumb flexion in combination with wrist ulnar deviation and/or palmar flexion.
- Use the power grip position when possible instead of using the thumb with any type of work or avocational activities.

S.F.M. Duncan and C.W. Flowers, *Therapy of the Hand and Upper Extremity: Rehabilitation Protocols*, DOI 10.1007/978-3-319-14412-2_62, © Springer International Publishing Switzerland 2015

- Incorporate more of the arm when turning nuts and bolts to distribute the overall force.
- Work with the wrist in a neutral position.

Discharge Criteria

- Patient is able to demonstrate proper tendon protection techniques.

Chapter 63
DeQuervain's Tenosynovitis Release

1 Week

- The bulky compressive dressing is removed and appropriate edema control is initiated.
- Active and passive ROM exercises are initiated 6 times a day for 10-min sessions to the thumb and wrist.
- Patient is able to perform finger eating.

2 Weeks

- Scar massage and manual desensitization exercises may be initiated within 24 h of suture removal.
- Patient is able to use hand as assist in dressing, bathing, and light hygiene.

3–4 Weeks

- Progressively return to normal use of the hand.
- Including strengthening program.
- Begin light household activities.

Discharge Criteria

- Independent in all ADLs including dressing, hygiene, and light housekeeping progressing to moderate housekeeping activities.
- Average number of visits—6.

S.F.M. Duncan and C.W. Flowers, *Therapy of the Hand and Upper Extremity: Rehabilitation Protocols*, DOI 10.1007/978-3-319-14412-2_63, © Springer International Publishing Switzerland 2015

Additional Comments

- In terms of patient education, advise the patient on the following:

  ○ Avoid thumb flexion in combination with ulnar deviation and/or palmar flexion.
  ○ Use the power grip position when possible instead of using the thumb with any type of work or vocational activities.
  ○ Incorporate more of the arm when turning nuts and bolts to distribute the overall force.
  ○ Work with the wrist in a neutral position.

- Once the patient is totally asymptomatic in the postoperative phase, protective splinting should not be necessary.

Chapter 64
Extensor Tendon Reposition for Rheumatoid Patients

Note: This procedure may often be performed in conjunction with other reconstructive procedures for the rheumatoid arthritis.

5–7 Days

- A wrist and MP block splint is fitted positioning the wrist in 15° of extension and the MPs in extension for continual wear.
- Active and passive ROM exercises are initiated to the IPs within the restraints of the splint.

3 Weeks

- A long dorsal outrigger is fitted positioning the wrist in 15° of extension and the MPs in 0° extension and neutral alignment.
- Composite active ROM exercises are initiated within the restraints of the LDO. Passive extension is allowed.
- The wrist and MP block splint is worn between exercise sessions and at night.

6 Weeks

- Active assistive (self-passive) ROM exercises are initiated.

S.F.M. Duncan and C.W. Flowers, *Therapy of the Hand and Upper Extremity: Rehabilitation Protocols*,
DOI 10.1007/978-3-319-14412-2_64,
© Springer International Publishing Switzerland 2015

7 Weeks

- Passive ROM exercises may be initiated as necessary.
- Dynamic flexion and splinting or taping may be initiated as necessary. However, taping is contraindicated for MP arthroplasty.

7–8 Weeks

- The LDO may be discontinued so long as there is a minimal extensor lag ($\leq 15°$).

8–10 Weeks

- The wrist and MP block splint is discontinued.

Discharge Criteria

Patient will be able to complete fastenings and light dressing activities.

Chapter 65
EPL Repair

0–3 Weeks

- Bulky compressive dressing.

2–4 Weeks

- The bulky dressing is removed.
- Edema control is initiated as needed.
- A wrist and thumb static splint with the wrist in 15° of extension and the thumb in full extension is fitted for continual wear.
- Initiate scar massage and remolding techniques.
- Initiate ROM of digits not splinted.
- No use of thumb for ADLs.

4 Weeks

- Active ROM exercises are initiated to the wrist and thumb each hour for a minimum of 6 times a day.
- The splint is continued between exercises and at night.
- Begin light pick up activities for eating.

6 Weeks

- Passive ROM exercises are initiated to the wrist and thumb each hour. Monitor for extensor lag at the IP level of the thumb.

S.F.M. Duncan and C.W. Flowers, *Therapy of the Hand and Upper Extremity: Rehabilitation Protocols*, DOI 10.1007/978-3-319-14412-2_65, © Springer International Publishing Switzerland 2015

- The splint may be gradually decreased or discontinued, if extensor lag is not present. If the extensor lag is limited at the IP joint, the splint may be adjusted to include the IP joint alone.
- Patient may use hand for bathing and dressing, with the exception of a static pinch.

7 Weeks

- Dynamic flexion splinting may be initiated as necessary to increase composite passive flexion of the thumb. If extensor lag is 15° or more, hold on dynamic flexion.

8 Weeks

- Gentle progressive strengthening may be initiated using a nerf ball, putty, and a hand helper.
- Resistive pinch activities are initiated.

Discharge Criteria

- Patient will be independent in all self-care activities and begin light household activities.

Chapter 66
FCU/FCR Tendonitis or FCR Tunnel Syndrome Nonoperative

Flexor Carpi Tendinitis or FCR Tunnel Syndrome

- 0–6 Weeks:

  ○ A wrist immobilization splint is applied in 10° of flexion and slight radial deviation for continual wear. Patients are generally reevaluated between 3 and 6 weeks. If symptoms persist, immobilization may be continued for an additional 4–6 weeks.

  ○ Gentle ROM and progressive strengthening of the hand is initiated after resolution of the acute symptoms.

  ○ *Note*: Pain is exacerbated by direct palpation, passive wrist extension, or resisted wrist flexor.

Flexor Carpi Ulnaris Tendinitis: Conservative Management

- 0–6 Weeks:

  ○ A wrist immobilization splint is applied in 10° of volar flexion and slight ulnar deviated for continual wear. Patients are generally reevaluated between 3 and 6 weeks. If the symptoms persist, splinting may be continued for an additional 4–6 weeks.

  ○ Gentle ROM and progressive strengthening of the hand is initiated after resolution of the acute symptoms.

S.F.M. Duncan and C.W. Flowers, *Therapy of the Hand and Upper Extremity: Rehabilitation Protocols*, DOI 10.1007/978-3-319-14412-2_66, © Springer International Publishing Switzerland 2015

- ○ *Note*: Instruct patient to attempt to minimize repetitive activities in which a significant degree of wrist ulnar deviation and palmar flexion is necessary.

Discharge Criteria

- Patient will be able to demonstrate the use of tendon protection techniques in basic ADLs.

Chapter 67
FPL Repair, Early Mobilization

0–5 Days

- Bulky compressive dressing.

3–5 Days

- The bulky compressive dressing is removed.
- Appropriate edema control is applied.
- A dorsal blocking splint is fitted to the wrist and thumb for continual wear with the wrist in 20° of palmar flexion, thumb MCP/IP in 15° of flexion at each hint, and thumb CMC in palmar abduction.
- Controlled passive mobilization is initiated every hour as stated in the handout "Home Exercise Program for Flexor Tendon Repair of the Thumb (initial 4½ weeks)."
- Once sutures are removed, scar management is initiated.

4½ Weeks

- The splint is removed every hour for the exercises as stated in the handout "Home Exercise Program for Flexor Tendon Repair of the Thumb (4½ weeks postoperatively)."
- The splint is continued between exercises and at night.

S.F.M. Duncan and C.W. Flowers, *Therapy of the Hand and Upper Extremity: Rehabilitation Protocols*, DOI 10.1007/978-3-319-14412-2_67,

5½ Weeks

- FES may be initiated to the FPL to increase tendon excursion.
- The dorsal blocking splint is discontinued.
- A wrist and thumb static splint is fitted to wear between exercises and at night to resolve any extrinsic flexor tightness.
- The exercise program is upgraded as stated in the handout "Home Exercise Program for Flexor Tendon Repair of the Thumb (5½ weeks postoperatively)."

6 Weeks

- Passive extension exercises are initiated to the thumb and wrist.

8 Weeks

- Gentle, progressive strengthening is initiated. Light grasp is allowed.
- No heavy lifting or heavy use of the hand is allowed.

10–12 Weeks

- May return to full use of the hand, including sports.

Discharge Criteria

- Independent in all pinching activities including turning key, pulling up pants, and writing.

Chapter 68
Opponensplasty (EIP to APB)

3 Weeks

- The bulky dressing is removed and appropriate edema control measures are initiated as necessary.
- A dorsal blocking splint is fitted positioning the wrist in 0° of palmar flexion with the thumb in wide palmar abduction for continual wear. Do not include the digits in the splint. (if the transfer is routed to the axis of the wrist, then the wrist should be positioned in 5° of extension versus palmar flexion. Review of the operative note and/or discussion with the surgeon should provide this information.)
- AROM and PROM exercises are initiated for 10 min sessions within the restrains off the dorsal blocking splint. Tendon transfer exercises are emphasized by attempting to independently extend the index finger while simultaneously bringing the thumb into opposition.
- Functional activities should be emphasized in which the patient must have wide palmar grasp.
- FES may be initiated to facilitate tendon excursion and muscle reeducation.
- Scar management techniques may be initiated.
- Patient may begin light pickup activities for eating, assist in dressing and bathing.

S.F.M. Duncan and C.W. Flowers, *Therapy of the Hand and Upper Extremity: Rehabilitation Protocols*, DOI 10.1007/978-3-319-14412-2_68, © Springer International Publishing Switzerland 2015

6 Weeks

• The dorsal blocking splint is discontinued.
• Active and passive ROM exercises are initiated for extension of the thumb and wrist. Exercises place emphasis on prehension tasks and wide palmar grasp.
• A web spacer splint may be fitted as necessary for protection.
• Patient may utilize hand for dressing, bathing, hygiene, and eating without resistance.

8 Weeks

• D/C the web spacer.
• Progressive strengthening may be initiated beginning with a nerf ball and progressing to a hand exerciser. In many cases, gently strengthening can begin at 6 weeks.
• Progressive resistive activities.

Discharge Criteria

• Patient will be independent in dressing, hygiene, eating, bathing, and progressive household activities.

Part XI
Hand/Finger Bone Injuries

Chapter 69
Arthrodesis MCP, PIP, or DIP

2 Weeks

- Once the bulky dressing is removed, edema control is initiated to the digit.
- A protective gutter splint and/or tip protector is applied to the fused joint for continual wear.
- Active and passive ROM exercises may be initiated to all uninvolved joints.
- The bases of the pins are cleaned daily with mercurochrome or hydrogen peroxide.
- If a screw or plates and screws used, begin desensitization to the incision site.
- Scar management may be initiated using scar massage with lotion, elastomer, or otoform.

6 Weeks

- Assuming the fusion is well-healed, the pin is removed by surgeon.
- The protective splinting is discontinued once the fusion is clinically healed as determined by the surgeon.

Discharge Criteria

- Independent self-care with difficulty.

S.F.M. Duncan and C.W. Flowers, *Therapy of the Hand and Upper Extremity: Rehabilitation Protocols*, DOI 10.1007/978-3-319-14412-2_69, © Springer International Publishing Switzerland 2015

Chapter 70
Bony Mallet Finger with Pinning

0–6 Weeks

- A tip protector splint is fitted to wear at all times allowing MCP and PIP ROM.
- The pin is cleaned with hydrogen peroxide daily.

6 Weeks

- The pin is pulled.
- AROM exercises are initiated to the DIP 10 min/h, six times a day.
- A mallet splint is continued between exercises and at night.

7 Weeks

- PROM exercises are initiated to the DIP joint, so long as there is minimal extensor lag.
- The splint is continued between exercises and at night.

8 Weeks

- The splint is decreased to night wear for 2 weeks and discontinued.
- Strengthening can be initiated.

Discharge Criteria

- Independent in all self-care tip pinch activities.

S.F.M. Duncan and C.W. Flowers, *Therapy of the Hand and Upper Extremity: Rehabilitation Protocols*,
DOI 10.1007/978-3-319-14412-2_70,
© Springer International Publishing Switzerland 2015

Chapter 71
Distal Phalanx or Tuft Fractures

0–1 Week

- A tip protector is applied for continual wear.

1 Week

- Active ROM exercises are initiated for 10 min/h, six times a day.
- The splint is continued between exercises and at night.
- Desensitization exercises are initiated.

3 Weeks

- PROM exercises may be initiated if fracture is clinically healed.
- The tip protector splint is continued PRN for protection.

4 Weeks

- Strengthening exercises may begin.

Discharge Criteria

- Independent in all self-care tip pinch activities.

S.F.M. Duncan and C.W. Flowers, *Therapy of the Hand and Upper Extremity: Rehabilitation Protocols*,
DOI 10.1007/978-3-319-14412-2_71,
© Springer International Publishing Switzerland 2015

Chapter 72
Dorsal PIP Fracture
or Dislocation Postoperative

5–7 Days

- Bulky compressive dressing is removed.
- A finger-based dorsal blocking splint with the PIP in 30° of flexion is fitted for continual wear.
- Active ROM exercises are initiated 10 min/h, six times a day.

2 Weeks

- Passive ROM exercises are initiated to the PIP joint and DIP joints within the splint.

3–6 Weeks

- The dorsal blocking splint is adjusted weekly to increase PIP extension 10° each week.

6 Weeks

- The dorsal blocking splint is discontinued.
- Active and passive ROM exercises are initiated every hour.
- Static or dynamic extension splinting is initiated PRN.

8 Weeks

- Strengthening is initiated.

S.F.M. Duncan and C.W. Flowers, *Therapy of the Hand and Upper Extremity: Rehabilitation Protocols*,
DOI 10.1007/978-3-319-14412-2_72,
© Springer International Publishing Switzerland 2015

Discharge Criteria

• Independent in self-care.

Chapter 73
Finger Amputation

3–5 Days

- Initiate wound care: dressings, whirlpool, and/or debridement.
- Apply light compressive dressings, ace wraps, or coban for edema control.
- Initiate active or active assistance ROM exercises to all upper extremity joints.
- TENS may be used PRN for pain.
- For digital level amputation, tip protector splints may be fitted to prevent additional trauma.

2 Weeks and/or Wound Closure

- Following suture removal (assuming the wounds are well healed) begin scar massage with lotion, or the use of otoform.
- Begin desensitization.
- Progressive strengthening may be initiated as appropriate for the level of amputation.
- Patient may begin ADLs as tolerated once the wound has closed.

Discharge Criteria

- Patient will be independent in dressing, eating, bathing, and light hygiene activities.

S.F.M. Duncan and C.W. Flowers, *Therapy of the Hand and Upper Extremity: Rehabilitation Protocols*,
DOI 10.1007/978-3-319-14412-2_73,
© Springer International Publishing Switzerland 2015

Chapter 74
Metacarpal Fracture Closed Reduction

0–3 Weeks

- Short arm cast with or without MCPs immobilized in approximately 50° of flexion.

3–4 Weeks

- Cast is removed if sufficient healing present.
- A wrist immobilization splint (for shaft or base fractures) or a safe position splint (for head or neck or distal shaft fractures) is fitted to wear between exercises and at night.
- Active and passive exercises are initiated to the IP joints.
- AROM only is initiated to the MCP joints.
- FES may be used to enhance tendon excursion.

6 Weeks

- PROM exercises may be initiated to the MCP joints.
- Dynamic splinting may be initiated to PRN to reduce joint or tendon tightness.
- The splint is continued for protection only between exercises and at night.

8 Weeks

- Gentle, progressive strengthening is initiated with putty and hand helper.
- Splint is discontinued.

S.F.M. Duncan and C.W. Flowers, *Therapy of the Hand and Upper Extremity: Rehabilitation Protocols*, DOI 10.1007/978-3-319-14412-2_74, © Springer International Publishing Switzerland 2015

Discharge Criteria

- Independent self-care activities.

Chapter 75
Metacarpal Fracture ORIF

3–7 Days

- Bulky dressing is removed.
- A wrist immobilization splint (for base fractures) or a safe position (for head/neck and distal shaft fractures) is fitted to wear between exercises and at night.
- AROM exercises are initiated to the MCP joint. Active and passive ROM exercises are initiated to the IP joints.

2 Weeks

- Scar management.

3 Weeks

- Passive ROM exercises are initiated to the MCP joints.
- Splint may be discontinued and buddy tapes used instead.
- May begin use for very light ADLs.

6 Weeks

- Gentle progressive strengthening is initiated.
- The splint or buddy tapes are discontinued.
- Resume normal activities.

Discharge Criteria

- Independent in self-care activities.

S.F.M. Duncan and C.W. Flowers, *Therapy of the Hand and Upper Extremity: Rehabilitation Protocols*,
DOI 10.1007/978-3-319-14412-2_75,
© Springer International Publishing Switzerland 2015

Chapter 76
Middle Phalanx Fracture Closed Reduction

0–3 Weeks

- Appropriate edema control measures are applied.
- A gutter splint with IP joints in full extension is applied for continual wear.

3 Weeks

- AROM exercises are initiated to the PIP and DIP joints 10 min/h.
- The splint is continued between exercises and at night.
- Scar management is initiated.
- FES may be initiated.

6 Weeks

- PROM exercises are initiated if the fracture is clinically healed.
- Dynamic splinting may be initiated.

8 Weeks

- Strengthening is initiated.
- Splint is discontinued.

Discharge Criteria

- Independent self-care.

S.F.M. Duncan and C.W. Flowers, *Therapy of the Hand and Upper Extremity: Rehabilitation Protocols*, DOI 10.1007/978-3-319-14412-2_76, © Springer International Publishing Switzerland 2015

Chapter 77
Middle Phalanx Fracture ORIF or External Fixation

0–1 Week

- Continue bulky compressive dressing.

1 Week

- Bulky compressive dressing is removed.
- Appropriate edema control is applied.
- A gutter with IP joints in full extension is fitted to wear between exercises and at night.
- AROM exercises are initiated 15 min/h.

2 Weeks

- Initiate scar management.

3 Weeks

- PROM exercises are initiated 15 min/h.
- The splint is continued between exercises and at night.
- Dynamic splinting may be initiated PRN.

6 Weeks

- Gentle, progressive strengthening is initiated.
- The splint may be discontinued if the fracture is clinically healed.

S.F.M. Duncan and C.W. Flowers, *Therapy of the Hand and Upper Extremity: Rehabilitation Protocols*,
DOI 10.1007/978-3-319-14412-2_77,
© Springer International Publishing Switzerland 2015

Discharge Criteria

- Independent self-care activities.

Chapter 78
MP Joint Implant Arthroplasty for Rheumatoid Patients (Four Digits)

3–5 Days

3 days if MP joint arthroplasty only; 5 days if multiple procedures performed in addition

- The bulky dressing is removed.
- A light compressive dressing is initiated along with digital level fingersocks or Coban. The dressing is changed each visit and worn until suture removal (14 days postoperation).
- An RA splint is fabricated for continual wear during the day. The hand is positioned in the splint as follows:

  o Wrist: 15° extension (*Note*: This may be adjusted to 0–15° of palmar flexion if there is an extensor lag at the MP level. By increasing wrist flexion, this assists with facilitating MP extension as the patient actively extends.)
  o MP joints: 0° of extension and neutral alignment with the rubber band traction. The slings are positioned such that there is approximately a 60° angle of radial pull from the outrigger to the proximal phalanx with the rubber band traction. The outrigger bar should be positioned directly above the proximal phalanx. Approximately 3 oz of tension is placed on the rubber band traction. Number 18 rubber bands are utilized.

S.F.M. Duncan and C.W. Flowers, *Therapy of the Hand and Upper Extremity: Rehabilitation Protocols*,
DOI 10.1007/978-3-319-14412-2_78,
© Springer International Publishing Switzerland 2015

It is important to ensure the MP joints *DO NOT HYPEREXTEND*, particularly the small finger, which is susceptible to this problem.

o Index MP joint: A "supinator" attachment is worn on the index finger between exercise sessions to protect the radial collateral ligament (RCL) reconstruction. The supinator bar is extended radially from the splint and is attached to the index finger using Velcro and a number 18 rubber band.

• An extension resting pan splint is fabricated to wear at night. The hand is positioned in the following manner:

o The digits are placed basically in full extension.

o The MP joints are held in neutral alignment to slight radial deviation.

o A "supinator" strap is applied to the index finger to prevent pronation of the finger.

• AROM exercises are initiated 15 min each hour. Range of motion exercises are performed with MP slings on the digits. Emphasis is placed on composite flexion, extension exercises, and isolated MP flexion. PROM exercises are initially performed two times a day (15 repetitions to each digit in a composite fashion, isolated MP, PIP, and DIP flexion). Patients which have limited passive MP flexion may increase passive range of motion up to 4–6 times a day, so long as an extensor lag is not significant (<30°). The passive range of motion exercises should be performed by the therapist with each patient visit back to therapy. It is important to begin with the small finger as it is the most likely to have limited passive flexion.

• Educate patient in joint protection for the nonsurgical hand.

1 Week

• Dynamic flexion may be initiated as needed if the MP extensor lag is less than 30° and the passive MP flexion is less than 75°. The dynamic flexion may be to the MP joints alone or compositely if there is some degree of extrinsic extensor tightness.

2 Weeks

- Begin scar massage once sutures are removed.

6 Weeks

- Light prehensile activities are permitted outside of the RA splint 3–4 times a day for approximately 15–30 min.

12 Weeks

- The RA splint, which is worn during the day, may be discontinued at this time. The extension resting pan splint is continued for a year.
- Soft putty or gentle restrictive exercises may be initiated to enhance the overall strength and thus, functional performance of the patient's hand.
- The patient's functional status should be reevaluated at this time. The patient should be provided with joint protection principles and energy conservation principles. In addition, the patient should be assessed for adaptive equipment needs.

Precautions

- Caution must be taken to avoid any lateral stress to the implant arthroplasty for 10–12 weeks (particularly to the index finger prosthesis).
- *DO NOT* attempt to gain passive flexion beyond 90°. This increases the risk of fracturing the prosthesis.

Discharge Criteria

- Patient should be able to demonstrate independence in fastening, bathing, and mini-mod assisting in dressing.

Chapter 79
MP Joint Implant Arthroplasty for Traumatic Injuries

1–3 Days

- The bulky dressing is removed.
- A light compressive dressing is applied to be worn for the initial 2 weeks postoperatively.
- A long dorsal outrigger splint is fitted with the rubber band traction from the outrigger positioning the MP joints in neutral alignment. The splint is worn continually throughout the day.
- Active range of motion exercises initiated 10 min each hour. The outrigger splint is worn during the active ROM exercises. Passive ROM exercises are initiated on an hourly basis as well. The rubber band traction is removed from the digits to perform the passive ROM exercises each hour. PROM to MCP, PIP, DIP, and composite.
- Dynamic flexion splinting may be initiated within the first week if passive flexion is less than 70° and there is an extensor lag less than 30°. (*Note*: It is usually necessary to add dynamic flexion splinting in the early postoperative days and it is not unusual for the patient to require a wearing schedule of 6 h a day or more.)
- An extension resting pain splint is fitted to wear at night to maintain correct alignment and neutral positioning of the MP joints.

S.F.M. Duncan and C.W. Flowers, *Therapy of the Hand and Upper Extremity: Rehabilitation Protocols*,
DOI 10.1007/978-3-319-14412-2_79,
© Springer International Publishing Switzerland 2015

  o *Note*: If only one digit is involved the digit may be buddy strapped eliminating the use of the outrigger splint.

6 Weeks

• Gentle, progressive strengthening may be initiated using a piece of foam, putty, or hand helper.
• Assuming the joints are in excellent alignment and quite stable, buddy taping may be initiated to an adjacent digit to allow light activity during the day. This allows the patient to be out of the outrigger during the day.

8–10 Weeks

• The long dorsal outrigger may be totally discontinued at this point in time. The extension resting pan splint is continued at night for approximately 3–4 months.

Precautions

• Caution must be taken to avoid any lateral stress to the implant arthroplasty for 8–10 weeks (particularly to the index finger prosthesis).
• Do not attempt to gain passive flexion beyond 90°. This increases the risk of fracturing the prosthesis.

Discharge Criteria

• Patient should be independent in all dressing activities, eating, and hygiene. Patient may begin light household activities.

Chapter 80
PIP Joint Implant Arthroplasty

1–3 Days

- The bulky dressing is removed and a light compressive dressing is applied to the hand and forearm. Digital level fingersocks are applied for edema control.
- A gutter splint is fitted, holding the digit in full extension to be worn between exercise sessions and at night. (*Note*: A full extension resting pan may be fitted if multiple joints are replaced.) The gutter splint may require high lateral side if there is any tendency for the joint to deviate from neutral alignment.
- Active ROM and passive range of motion exercises are initiated four times a day for 10 min sessions. The patient is cautioned against any lateral stress to the digit(s).
- If there is any lateral deviation at the PIP joint a "bowling alley" splint may be used to control any lateral joint motion as the patient performs the active range of motion exercises.

***With erosive osteoarthritis, the joints will frequently become swollen and inflamed following surgery. Therefore, it may be necessary to be less aggressive in the initial postoperative days by limiting the exercise sessions to three times a day, with emphasis on digital level edema control.

S.F.M. Duncan and C.W. Flowers, *Therapy of the Hand and Upper Extremity: Rehabilitation Protocols*, DOI 10.1007/978-3-319-14412-2_80, © Springer International Publishing Switzerland 2015

- Coban is not recommended for the digit with postoperative edema. With the spiral wrapping of the coban, it may create a torsional force on the PIP joint and affect the stability of the prosthesis.

5–7 Days

- Dorsal taping or dynamic flexion splinting may be initiated if passive flexion is less than 70° and there is an extensor lag less than or equal to 30°. (*Note*: IP taping is discouraged so as to avoid torsional forces to the PIP joint.)
- Exercises may be increased to every 2 h as needed. This is somewhat dependent on the degree of extensor lag at the PIP level and the amount of flexion.

3 Weeks

- Begin interval splinting.

8 Weeks

- Gentle progressive strengthening may be initiated with a small nerf ball and progressing to putty.
- The patient should gradually be weaned out of the gutter splint at this time. This splint should be completely discontinued between 12 and 14 weeks.

Additional Comments

- An average arc of motion at the PIP joint is 60–70°. There is generally an extensor lag of ±15°, with PIP joint flexion ranging between 75 and 85°.
- Caution must be taken to avoid lateral stress to the digit for a minimum of 10–12 weeks postoperatively.
- Do not attempt to gain passive flexion beyond 90° as this may increase the risk of fracturing the prosthesis.

Discharge Criteria

- Patient is able to dress, eat, bathe, and complete light hygiene activities independently.

Chapter 81
PIP Joint Implant Arthroplasty for Traumatic Injuries

2–4 Days

- The bulky dressing is removed and a light compressive dressing is applied to the hand and forearm. Digital level fingersocks are applied for digital level edema control.
- An extension gutter splint, with well-molded lateral sides is fitted to wear at all times between exercises and at night.
- Active range of motion and passive range of motion exercises are initiated six times a day for 10 min sessions. This may need to be increased to every hour within the initial week of therapy in order to maximize the PIP joint flexion. AROM with buddy straps.
- The patient is cautioned against any lateral stress to the digit.
- If there is any lateral deviation of the digit a "bowling alley" splint may be fabricated to control the lateral joint motion as the patient exercises.

5–7 Days

- Dorsal taping and dynamic flexion splinting may be initiated to increase passive flexion of the PIP joint. This is often necessary with PIP joint implant arthroplasties for traumatic injuries. In an attempt to increase passive flexion, it is important to monitor the extensor lag at the PIP joint and ensure that the extensor lag is minimized (less than 25°).

S.F.M. Duncan and C.W. Flowers, *Therapy of the Hand and Upper Extremity: Rehabilitation Protocols*,
DOI 10.1007/978-3-319-14412-2_81,
© Springer International Publishing Switzerland 2015

- *Note*: IP taping is discouraged so as to avoid any torsional forces to the PIP joint.

8 Weeks

- Gentle, progressive strengthening may be initiated using a nerf ball and putty.
- The patient should gradually be weaned out of the gutter splint by 10–12 weeks. This is primarily determined by the lateral stability of the PIP joint, as well as, the degree of extensor lag at the PIP level.

Precaution

- Caution must be taken to avoid lateral stress to the digit for a minimum of 10–12 weeks postoperatively.
- Do not attempt passive flexion beyond 90° as this will increase the risk of fracturing the prosthesis.
- Coban is not recommended for the digit with postoperative edema. The coban may create torsional force on the Pip joint and affect the stability of the prosthesis.
- *Note*: An interesting observation with PIP joint implant arthroplasties is that the PIP joint extension is often 5° less than the preoperative PIP extension and the flexion generally reaches 75–85°.

Discharge Criteria

- Patient is able to dress, eat, bathe, and complete light hygiene activities independently.

Chapter 82
Proximal Phalanx Fracture Closed Reduction

0–3 Weeks

- A splint or cast is applied holding the digits in a safe position.

3 Weeks

- The cast is removed if sufficient healing is present.
- AROM exercises are initiated to the digits and wrist 10 min/h.
- A safe position splint (midshaft/base fractures) or a gutter splint (for neck/head fractures) is fitted to wear between exercises and at night.
- Begin scar management if needed.

4 Weeks

- FES may be initiated to enhance tendon excursion.

6 Weeks

- If fracture is clinically healed:
- PROM exercises are initiated 10 min/h.
- Dynamic splinting may be initiated PRN.
- Patient wearing a safe position splint may have it reduced to a gutter given good MCP ROM.
- Light ADLs can be initiated.

S.F.M. Duncan and C.W. Flowers, *Therapy of the Hand and Upper Extremity: Rehabilitation Protocols*, DOI 10.1007/978-3-319-14412-2_82, © Springer International Publishing Switzerland 2015

8 Weeks

- The splint is discontinued.
- Gentle, progressive strengthening is initiated.
- Normal light activities are initiated.

Discharge Criteria

- Independent in self-care.

Chapter 83
Proximal Phalanx Fracture ORIF

0–1 Week

- Bulky compressive dressing with the digits in safe position.

3 Days–1 Week

- Bulky compressive dressing is removed.
- AROM exercises are initiated to the digits 10 min/h.
- Appropriate edema control measures are applied.
- A safe position splint (for midshaft/base fractures) or a gutter splint (for neck/head fractures) is fitted to wear between exercises and at night.
- Dynamic flexion splinting may be initiated as necessary to increase PROM in flexion. Monitor for extensor lag.

2 Weeks

- Begin scar management.

3 Weeks

- PROM exercises are initiated 15 min/h.
- Dynamic splinting may be initiated PRN.
- Splint is continued between exercises and at night.
- Patient with good AROM may use buddy tapes and reduce use of the safe position splint.

S.F.M. Duncan and C.W. Flowers, *Therapy of the Hand and Upper Extremity: Rehabilitation Protocols*, DOI 10.1007/978-3-319-14412-2_83, © Springer International Publishing Switzerland 2015

4–6 Weeks

- Gentle, progressive strengthening is initiated.
- The splint may be discontinued if the fracture is clinically healed.
- Begin light ADLs.

8 Weeks

- Normal use.

Discharge Criteria

- Independent in self-care.

Chapter 84
Volar PIP Fracture or Dislocation Postoperative

1 Week

- Bulky compressive dressing is removed.
- A gutter splint is fitted with the PIP joint at neutral for continual wear.
- Active and passive ROM exercises are initiated to the MCP and DIP joints 10 min/h, six times a day. No motion is allowed to the PIP joint.

6 Weeks

- AROM exercises are initiated to the PIP joint.
- The splint is continued between exercises and at night.

8 Weeks

- PROM exercises are initiated to the PIP joint.
- Dynamic splinting is initiated PRN.
- Gentle strengthening is initiated.
- Extension splint is gradually decreased as long as extension lag is not present.

  ***Note*: The initiation of PROM and/or dynamic flexion splinting should be delayed if an extension lag greater than or equal to 30° is present.

S.F.M. Duncan and C.W. Flowers, *Therapy of the Hand and Upper Extremity: Rehabilitation Protocols*,
DOI 10.1007/978-3-319-14412-2_84,
© Springer International Publishing Switzerland 2015

Part XII
Hand/Finger Nerve Injuries

Chapter 85
Complex Regional Pain Syndrome (CRPS)

- Therapy for CRPS should address the areas of edema, pain, hypersensitivity, and ROM.
- Treatment should be kept within the patient's pain tolerance at all times.

Edema

- Edema control should be initiated which may consist of:

    o Elevation light compressing dressing.
    o An isotoner glove.
    o Jobst garment, or elastic stockinettes.
    o Fingersocks or Coban.
    o In addition, retrograde massage and gentle ROM exercises may assist in edema control.

Pain Management

- Treatment modalities which may be effective in managing the abnormal pain pattern include:

    o High or low rate TENS
    o Massage
    o Manual desensitization exercises

S.F.M. Duncan and C.W. Flowers, *Therapy of the Hand and Upper Extremity: Rehabilitation Protocols*,
DOI 10.1007/978-3-319-14412-2_85,
© Springer International Publishing Switzerland 2015

Splinting

- Patients are generally splinted in a safe position splint to wear between exercise sessions and at night.
- The purpose of the splint is to avoid the pain reflex position of MP flexion and IP flexion and to avoid joint contractures in the same position.
- Static and dynamic splinting may be initiated to enhance overall ROM of the wrist, fingers, and thumb as necessary. It is important that the static and dynamic splinting be within the patients comfort level.

ROM Exercises

- Active and gentle passive ROM exercises may be initiated. It is particularly important to exercise within the patients comfort level. Exercises should include ROM to the neck, shoulder girdle, elbow, forearm, wrist, and hand regardless of the level at which the problem is present with the dystrophy.
- As the patient's pain begins to subside somewhat, ROM exercises along with static and dynamic splinting may be increasingly aggressive.

Strengthening

- Strengthening may be initiated so long as edema is at a minimum and it does not increase the patient's level of pain.

Modalities

- It is important to not use whirlpools or heat modalities as an adjunct to the therapy program for patients with RSD.
- With these patients they have abnormal vasomotor response and therefore the use of heat modalities simply magnifies the problem.

Activities of Daily Living

- Begin light activities as tolerated such as finger eating, bathing, applying lotion and as assist in dressing.

Additional Comments

- Physicians may choose to use stellate ganglion blocks or possibly the gaunethidine blocks as an adjunct to therapy. In addition, elavil and prolixin may be considered as an antianxiety and antidepressant medications.

Chapter 86
Digital Nerve Repair

2 Weeks

- The bulky dressing is removed. Edema control is initiated consisting of fingersocks or Coban.
- A dorsal blocking splint is fitted to the involved digit in 30° of flexion at the PIP joint for continual wear, assuming the repair is near the PIP level or slightly distal to this point.
- *Note*: If the digital nerve is repaired near the MP level, the dorsal blocking gutter splint should include the MP joint along, positioning it in approximately 30° of flexion.
- Active and passive ROM exercises are initiated six times a day within the restraints of the dorsal blocking gutter.
- Scar massage with lotion and/or the use of otoform may be initiated within 24 h following suture removal.
- The patients may use their hand for light pickups within constraints of the splint.

3–6 Weeks

- The dorsal blocking gutter splint is adjusted into extension 10° each week until at neutral by 6 weeks. (Week 4 = 20°, Week 5 = 10°, Week 6 = 0°)
- The patients may use their hand for light activities, to assist in dressing.

S.F.M. Duncan and C.W. Flowers, *Therapy of the Hand and Upper Extremity: Rehabilitation Protocols*,
DOI 10.1007/978-3-319-14412-2_86,
© Springer International Publishing Switzerland 2015

6 Weeks

- The dorsal blocking splint is discontinued.
- Passive extension may be initiated to all joints.
- Extension splinting may be initiated if passive extension is limited. Generally it is not necessary to fabricate extension splints as the patient will generally recapture the extension.
- Progressive strengthening may be initiated at this time.

Discharge Criteria

- Independent in all dressing, eating, and hygiene activities. Begin use of hand in light housekeeping activities progressing to moderate.

Additional Comments

- Sensory reeducation is generally initiated between 8 and 10 weeks post repair. It is generally initiated when there is some sign of sensory return (protective sensation.)
- The dorsal blocking splint may have initially been fitted in greater flexion at either MP or PIP joint level if the digital nerve is repaired under greater degrees of tension.

Part XIII
Hand/Finger Soft Tissue/Ligament Injuries

.

Chapter 87
Boutonniere Deformity Nonoperative

ACUTE: Defined as one which occurs within 3 weeks of injury and in which full passive extension is passive.

- **0–6 Weeks**

    - A gutter splint or cylinder cast in full extension is applied to the PIP joint for continual wear. When changing the cast, do not allow any PIP flexion.
    - Active and passive ROM exercises are initiated to the MCP and DIP joints only.
    - Patient is not permitted to use digit for ADLs.

- **6 Weeks**

    - Active ROM exercises are initiated to the PIP joint. The splint is worn between exercises and at night.
    - Patient may begin to use hand for light pickup.

- **7 Weeks**

    - Passive ROM exercises are initiated PRN to the PIP joint. If an extensor lag begins to develop, then decrease passive flexion and/or limit exercise sessions.

- **8 Weeks**

    - Initiate gentle strengthening.
    - Patient is able to use hand for dressing, bathing, hygiene, and eating.

S.F.M. Duncan and C.W. Flowers, *Therapy of the Hand and Upper Extremity: Rehabilitation Protocols*, DOI 10.1007/978-3-319-14412-2_87, © Springer International Publishing Switzerland 2015

- **Discharge Criteria**

    - Independent in all self-care activities.
    - Average number of visits—8.

CHRONIC: Defined as longer than 3 weeks old: full passive extension is usually not present.

- **Initial Treatment**

    - Full passive PIP extension must be achieved with dynamic and/or serial casting, static splinting.
    - When passive extension is to neutral, a cylinder cast or boutonniere gutter splint is fitted for continual wear.
    - No use of the digit is permitted without the splint.

- **0–8 Weeks**

    - The PIP joint is held at 0° continually with a gutter or cylinder cast.
    - Active and passive ROM exercises are initiated to the MCP and DIP joints only.
    - No use of the digit is permitted without the splint.

- **8 Weeks**

    - Active and gentle, passive ROM exercises are initiated to the PIP joint.
    - The splint is worn between exercises and at night.
    - Patient may begin light eating, bathing, and dressing activities.

- **9 Weeks**

    - Taping or dynamic splinting may be initiated PRN to increase ROM.
    - Strengthening is initiated PRN.

- **Discharge Criteria**

    - Independent in all self-care activities.

Chapter 88
Pulley Repair or Reconstruction

0–8 Weeks

- Remove bulky dressing within first 2 weeks.
- Apply circumferential pressure dressing to the repaired pulley site.
- The method for creating the circumferential pressure is generally either one half inch paper tape or utilizing a pulley ring with a low temperature forming thermoplastic such as polyform.
- The purpose of the circumferential support is to prevent disruption or attenuation, "stretching out," of the pulley reconstruction/repair.
- Wear the pulley tape or pulley ring continuously for 6–8 weeks.

Discharge Criteria

- Patient should be independent in all ADLs except that the patient may not use hand for lifting over 1 lb and no resistive gripping or pulling.

S.F.M. Duncan and C.W. Flowers, *Therapy of the Hand and Upper Extremity: Rehabilitation Protocols*, DOI 10.1007/978-3-319-14412-2_88, © Springer International Publishing Switzerland 2015

Chapter 89
Radial/Ulnar Collateral Ligament Repair/ Reconstruction of the Digital MP Joint

3 Weeks

- The bulky compressive dressing is removed and edema control measures are initiated as needed.
- A gutter splint, securing the MP joint in slight flexion (30°), is fitted to be worn between exercises and at night.
- AROM exercises are initiated six times a day for 10 min sessions. Buddy tapes are worn around the proximal phalanx of the injured digit and an adjacent digit during the exercise session.

6 Weeks

- PROM exercises may be initiated.
- The splint is continued for protection and comfort as desired. Buddy tapes may be used as an alternative method of protection.

8 Weeks

- The splint or buddy tapes are discontinued.
- Progressive strengthening may be initiated.

S.F.M. Duncan and C.W. Flowers, *Therapy of the Hand and Upper Extremity: Rehabilitation Protocols*, DOI 10.1007/978-3-319-14412-2_89, © Springer International Publishing Switzerland 2015

Chapter 90
Radial/Ulnar Collateral Ligament Repair/ Reconstruction of the PIP Joint

0–2 Weeks

- Continue bulky compressive dressing.

2–3 Weeks

- A gutter splint is fitted to be worn at all times.

3 Weeks

- Active ROM exercises are initiated 15 min/h using buddy tapes for the injured digit and adjacent digit.
- The splint is continued between exercises and at night.
- Patient should be independent in light hygiene activities and using hand as assist in dressing.

6 Weeks

- Passive ROM exercises are initiated.
- The splint is continued for protection and comfort.

8 Weeks

- The splint is discontinued.
- Gentle strengthening is initiated.
- Patient is able to complete all light activities, with progressive resistance.

S.F.M. Duncan and C.W. Flowers, *Therapy of the Hand and Upper Extremity: Rehabilitation Protocols*, DOI 10.1007/978-3-319-14412-2_90, © Springer International Publishing Switzerland 2015

Discharge Criteria

- Able to lift a carton of milk and sauce pan.
- Independent in all self-care activities.

Chapter 91
Radial/Ulnar Collateral Ligament Repair/ Reconstruction of the Thumb MP Joint

3 Weeks

- The bulky compressive dressing is removed and the MP joint pin is removed (if a pin has been utilized to stabilize the MP joint postoperatively).
- Initiate edema control.
- A wrist and thumb static splint is fitted for continual wear.
- Begin scar massage.

6 Weeks

- Active and gentle PROM exercises are initiated for 10 min sessions each hour.
- Care must be taken to avoid any lateral stress to the MP joint.
- Dynamic splinting may be initiated to increase PROM of the thumb.
- The wrist and thumb static splint is continued between exercises and at night for comfort and protection.
- Patient may begin light pickups for eating and object manipulation.

8 Weeks

- The splint may be discontinued.
- Progressive strengthening may be initiated.

S.F.M. Duncan and C.W. Flowers, *Therapy of the Hand and Upper Extremity: Rehabilitation Protocols*, DOI 10.1007/978-3-319-14412-2_91,
© Springer International Publishing Switzerland 2015

- Patient should be able to pull up pants and pull on socks.
- Patient is able to cut food with a knife and fork.

12 Weeks

- The patient may return to normal, unrestricted use of the involved hand.

***Note: Until this 12 week point it is valuable to continue the wrist and thumb static splint or a short opponens splint for heavy lifting and/or sports-related activities.

Discharge Criteria

- Independent in all activities requiring resistive pinch, such as turning key in ignition, opening packages, and turning knobs.

Chapter 92
Radial/Ulnar Collateral Ligament Strain of the Digital MCP Joint with Stretching of the Volar Plate

0–3 Weeks

- A hand-based safe position splint including the MP joints only is fitted to the involved digits for continual wear.
- Generally, the injured digit is secured to an adjacent digit in the safe position splint.
- Initiate edema control as needed.
- No use of hand for ADLs except with splint on.

3 Weeks

- The splint is discontinued as long as the patient is asymptomatic and non-painful at the site of the collateral ligament strain.
- AROM exercises may be initiated 6–8 times a day for 10-min sessions.
- *Passive extension of MP joint is not allowed at this time.*
- Patient is able to eat and use hand as assist in dressing.

6 Weeks

- Passive extension may be initiated to the MP joint.

8 Weeks

- If the patient is asymptomatic, begin progressive strengthening.

S.F.M. Duncan and C.W. Flowers, *Therapy of the Hand and Upper Extremity: Rehabilitation Protocols*, DOI 10.1007/978-3-319-14412-2_92, © Springer International Publishing Switzerland 2015

- Patient should be independent in all ADLs except progressive resistive grip and lifting activities.

***Note*: Patients may remain in safe position splint for longer duration of time initially if the discomfort secondary to the collateral ligament strain is persistent.

Modalities

- Iontophoresis has proven to be beneficial with some patients recovering from the pain and discomfort associated with collateral ligament strains. When iontophoresis is utilized, four (4) treatments are given on an every other day basis.

Discharge Criteria

- Independent in all ADLs.

Chapter 93
Radial/Ulnar Collateral Ligament Strain of the Thumb MCP Joint

0–3 Weeks

- A short opponens splint is fitted with the thumb in palmar abduction for continual wear.
- No activities allowed without splint.

3–6 Weeks

- The discomfort associated with the collateral ligament strain is reevaluated at this time. If the discomfort has decreased significantly then active and gentle PROM exercises may be initiated.
- The splint is continued for comfort and protection between exercise sessions.
- Patient should be able to pull clothing on and utilize a lateral pinch without complaints of pain.

8 Weeks

- Assuming the patient is asymptomatic the splint may be discontinued except for heavy lifting, resistive pinching, or for sports activities.
- Progressive strengthening may be initiated as needed.

Note: It is important to ensure that there remains good stability of the joint and that the discomfort for the collateral ligament strain is resolved before beginning an aggressive exercise program.

S.F.M. Duncan and C.W. Flowers, *Therapy of the Hand and Upper Extremity: Rehabilitation Protocols*, DOI 10.1007/978-3-319-14412-2_93, © Springer International Publishing Switzerland 2015

Modalities

• Iontophoresis has proven to be somewhat beneficial in assisting in quieting the discomfort associated with collateral ligament strains.

    ○ When initiated with this type of injury it is recommended that the patient receive four treatments on an every other day basis.

Discharge Criteria

• Patient is independent and pain free in all nonresistive pinching activities.
• Patient is able to manage use of thumb in resistive activities.

Chapter 94
Subtotal Palmar Fasciectomy for Dupuytren's Contracture

0–5 Days

- The bulky dressing is removed.
- Appropriate edema control is applied.
- Active and passive ROM exercises are initiated 6 times a day for 15 min sessions.
- An extension splint is fitted for the digits involved and worn between exercises and at night.
- Functional electrical stimulation (FES) may be used PRN to enhance tendon excursion.
- Dynamic splinting may be used PRN.
- Wound care is also initiated if patient underwent an open palm technique including whirlpool.

2 Weeks

- A silicone insert (otoform) is applied to splint if all wounds are healed to help minimize hypertrophic scarring and the patient has minimal edema. Initiate scar massage.
- Splint may be modified to a hand-based splint.
- A dynamic extension splint may be used during the day to facilitate extension.
- Use hand for bathing assist in ADLs once wound is healed.

S.F.M. Duncan and C.W. Flowers, *Therapy of the Hand and Upper Extremity: Rehabilitation Protocols*,
DOI 10.1007/978-3-319-14412-2_94,
© Springer International Publishing Switzerland 2015

4 Weeks

- The extension splint may be gradually decreased to 2–3 times a day to night wear only if the patient is able to maintain full active extension.
- Strengthening can be initiated once pain and edema have decreased.
- Patient should be independent in use of hand for eating, fastening, dressing, bathing, and hygiene.
- If scar continues to be sensitive initiate scar desensitization.

6–8 Weeks

- Strengthening may be initiated.
- Night splinting should continue for 6–12 months postoperatively at night.

Discharge Criteria

- Patient should be independent in all self-care activities and have begun return to light household activities.

Chapter 95
Trigger Finger Release

5 Days

- The bulky dressing is removed.
- Edema control is applied PRN.
- Active and passive ROM exercises are initiated to the digit 10 min/h.
- An extension gutter splint is fitted to include the MP, PIP, and DIP joints if digits are painful and/or edematous.
- Utilize Functional Electrical Stimulation (FES) as needed to facilitate tendon pull.

2 Weeks

- Scar massage and otoform are initiated.
- Patient should be able to perform light eating and dressing activities.
- Begin light rolling activities.

4–6 Weeks

- Gentle strengthening initiated with putty.
- Record continuous and repetitive grasping and releasing of the hand for long periods of time.
- Patient is independent in dressing, hygiene, and light household activities.

S.F.M. Duncan and C.W. Flowers, *Therapy of the Hand and Upper Extremity: Rehabilitation Protocols*, DOI 10.1007/978-3-319-14412-2_95,
© Springer International Publishing Switzerland 2015

Discharge Criteria

- Patient will be independent in dressing, eating, hygiene, and light-to-moderate household activities.

Part XIV
Hand/Finger Tendon Injuries

Chapter 96
Active Tendon Implant

Stage I

Day 1

- Dorsal blocking splint (DBS) with wrist at 30° flex, MP joints at 70°, and IP joints in full extension.
- Appropriate edema control methods are applied.
- Patient begins "passive hold exercises." ten repetitions 3–4 times a day.

  ○ "Passive hold exercises":

    (a) Patient relaxes forearm muscles and then uses his opposite hand to gently press his finger into flexion.
    (b) Patient then tries to hold the finger in that position with his own muscle power.
    (c) Have the patient use the most gentle muscle contraction possible.
    (d) Do 2 sets, patient pushes the finger in mid-flexion and one into complete flexion.
    (e) Following passive flexion, the patient actively extends the finger in the DBS.

Week 2

- If the patient begins to glide the tendon very early and excellent tendon pull-through is demonstrated, add an elastic band traction.

S.F.M. Duncan and C.W. Flowers, *Therapy of the Hand and Upper Extremity: Rehabilitation Protocols*,
DOI 10.1007/978-3-319-14412-2_96,
© Springer International Publishing Switzerland 2015

- Continue the passive hold exercise; add gentle passive flexion at this time.
- Begin scar management once the sutures are removed.

Week 6

- The DBS is removed and a wristlet and elastic band is applied.
- Continue passive hold exercises.
- Allow wrist extension only to neutral.

Week 8–10

- Patient may begin active ROM and discontinue use of wristlet.

Week 11

- Begin progressive resistive strengthening.

Week 12–14

- Full activities with power grip.
  ** In case of pulley reconstruction:
- Construct a Velcro and felt ring device to protect the repair. When edema decreases, a thermoplastic ring can be fabricated. Protect for 6 months.

Stage II: Following Tendon Graft

Day 1

- Apply dorsal blocking splint in wrist 30°, MP is at 70° and IP's full extension. Utilize early mobilization with elastic traction.
- Have the patient actively extend the digit and relax it allowing the elastic band to flex the finger. Patient completes this 10 times every hour.
- Gentle PROM is completed 6 times a day. Use appropriate edema control.
- Begin scar management once suture is removed.

Week 6–8

- Wristlet is applied with elastic traction.
- If patient has early pain-free gliding at 6 weeks, extend the period before you begin the wristlet and each of the next time tables.

Week 8–10

- Begin AROM and discontinue the wristlet.

Week 10–13

- Progressive strengthening is begun.

Chapter 97
Extensor Tendon Injury Zones 1 and 2 Nonoperative

Acute (<3 Weeks Old)

0–6 Weeks

- A volar mallet splint holding the DIP joint in 0–15° of hyperextension is fitted for continual wear. The splint should be removed once daily while holding the DIP in extension to allow air to the skin. The DIP joint should not be allowed to flex. If the finger appears very swollen, have the patient return for splint adjustments as needed.
- Patient may use hand for ADLs with splint on.

6 Weeks

- Active ROM exercises are initiated to the DIP joint 10 min/six times a day.
- The mallet splint is continued between exercises and at night.
- Patient may perform light gripping activities.

7 Weeks

- Passive ROM exercises are initiated to the DIP joint 10 min/six times a day.
- If the DIP extensor lag is present, then passive exercise may be discontinued.
- The mallet splint is continued between exercises and at night.

S.F.M. Duncan and C.W. Flowers, *Therapy of the Hand and Upper Extremity: Rehabilitation Protocols*, DOI 10.1007/978-3-319-14412-2_97, © Springer International Publishing Switzerland 2015

8 Weeks

- Gentle, progressive strengthening is initiated PRN.
- The mallet splint is gradually decreased and discontinued if an extensor lag is not present.

Chronic (>3 Weeks Old)

0–8 Weeks

- A mallet splint is fitted holding the DIP joint in 0–15° of hyperextension for continual wear.
- Active and passive ROM exercises are initiated to the MCP and PIP joints PRN.
- Patient may use hand for daily activities with splint on.

8 Weeks

- Active exercises are initiated to the DIP joint 10 min/six times a day.
- The mallet splint is continued between exercises and at night.

9 Weeks

- Passive ROM exercises are initiated to the DIP joint 10 min/six times a day.
- The mallet splint may be gradually decreased and then discontinued if an extensor lag is not present.
- Gentle, progressive strengthening is initiated PRN.

Discharge Criteria

- Patient will be independent in all self-care activities.

Chapter 98
Extensor Tendon Repair Zones 3 and 4

Anatomical structures potentially involved: Triangular ligament, lateral bands, central slip, and extensor hood.

0–2 Weeks

- Maintain bulky compressive dressing.

2–4 Weeks

- Bulky dressing is removed; edema control is initiated as needed.
- A gutter splint is fitted holding the PIP joint in full extension for continual wear.
- Begin scar massage once sutures are removed and apply otoform as needed.
- Patient may use hand for daily activities with splint on.

4 Weeks

- Active ROM exercises are initiated six times a day to the PIP joint, along with composite ROM of the entire digit.
- The splint is continued between exercises and at night.

6 Weeks

- Passive ROM exercises are initiated to the PIP joint if the extensor lag is <20°.

S.F.M. Duncan and C.W. Flowers, *Therapy of the Hand and Upper Extremity: Rehabilitation Protocols*, DOI 10.1007/978-3-319-14412-2_98,
© Springer International Publishing Switzerland 2015

- Taping and/or dynamic flexion splinting may be initiated PRN to increase ROM. Monitor for development of extensor lag.
- The gutter splint is gradually decreased to night wear if there is minimal extensor lag ($\leq 15°$).

8 Weeks

- Gentle, progressive strengthening is initiated PRN.
- The gutter splint is discontinued if an extensor lag is not present.

Discharge Criteria

- Patient is independent in all daily self-care activities.

Chapter 99
Extensor Tendon Repair Zones 5 and 6

Anatomical structures potentially involved: sagittal band, EDC, EIP, EDQM

0–2 Weeks

- Bulky compressive dressing.

2–3 Weeks

- The bulky dressing is removed.
- Edema control is initiated PRN.
- A wrist and P1 block is fitted holding the MCPs in 10–15° of flexion and the wrist in 30° of extension for continual wear.
- Active ROM to the IP joints is initiated within the constraints of the splint.
- Scar massage/retraction and scar remodeling are initiated to minimize adhesions.

4 Weeks

- Active ROM exercises are initiated to the wrist and digits out of the splint 10 min/h.
- FES or electrical stimulation may be used PRN to increase tendon excursion.
- The wrist and P1 block splint is continued between exercises and at night.

S.F.M. Duncan and C.W. Flowers, *Therapy of the Hand and Upper Extremity: Rehabilitation Protocols*, DOI 10.1007/978-3-319-14412-2_99, © Springer International Publishing Switzerland 2015

• Isolated EDC exercises are emphasized, as well as compo-
sition flexion and extension.

6 Weeks

• Passive flexion exercises are initiated to the wrist and
digits.
• Taping and/or dynamic flexion may be initiated PRN to
increase passive ROM.
• The wrist and P1 block splint is continued between exercises and at night.

7–8 Weeks

• The splint is decreased or discontinued if there are minimal
extensor lags ($\leq 15^\circ$).
• Gentle, progressive strengthening may be initiated for
both flexors and extensors.

   ○ *Note*: Hold on PROM and/or dynamic flexion splinting
   if extensor lags 25° are present. If the MP extensor lags
   are greater than 20° it is recommended to decrease
   exercise sessions to 4–6 times a day.

Discharge Criteria

• Patient is independent in all self-care, eating, dressing, and
light household activities.

Chapter 100
Extensor Tendon Repair Zones 7 and 8

Anatomical structures potentially involved: EPL, EPB, APL, EIP, ECU, ECRB, ECRL, EDC, and EDQM.

0–3 Weeks

- Bulky compressive dressing.

2–3 Weeks

- The bulky dressing is removed.
- Edema control is initiated as needed.
- A wrist and P1 block is fitted holding the MCPs in 10–15° of flexion and the wrist in 30° of extension for continual wear.
- Active and passive ROM exercises are initiated to the IP joints within the constraints of the splints.
- Scar massage and scar remolding techniques are utilized once sutures are removed.
- Patient is not permitted any use of hand.

4 Weeks

- Active ROM exercises are initiated to the wrist and digits 10 min/h.
- Scar massage/retraction and scar remodeling techniques are utilized to remodel tissue.
- The splint is continued between exercises and at night.

S.F.M. Duncan and C.W. Flowers, *Therapy of the Hand and Upper Extremity: Rehabilitation Protocols*, DOI 10.1007/978-3-319-14412-2_100, © Springer International Publishing Switzerland 2015

- FES or electrical stimulation may be used PRN to increase tendon excursion.
- Patient may begin light pickups.

6 Weeks

- Passive flexion exercises are initiated to the wrist and digits.
- The splint is continued between exercises and at night.
- Taping and/or dynamic flexion can be initiated to increase the composite passive flexion of the digits. Monitor for extensor lag.

7 Weeks

- The splint may be decreased or discontinued if significant extensor lags are not present. If the lag is 25° continue with MP block.
- Strengthening is initiated to flexors and extensors.
- *Note*: Extrinsic extensor tightness is generally significant.

Discharge Criteria

- Patient is independent in all self-care, eating, dressing, and light household activities.

Chapter 101
Extensor Tenolysis (With Dorsal PIP and MP Capsulectomy)

Day 1

- The bulky dressing is removed.
- Appropriate edema control is applied (it is important to monitor edema on the dorsum of the hand).
- Active and passive ROM exercises are initiated hourly for 10 min sessions. One exercise which is important to emphasize is passive MP flexion along with active IP extension. In addition, it is important to emphasize active MP extension with the IPs flexed for EDC excursion.
- A wrist immobilization splint with dynamic flexion to the MP joints along with extension gutters to the PIP and DIP joint is fitted to wear between exercise sessions during the day.
- A safe position splint is fabricated to wear at night.
- A composite dynamic flexion splint is fitted to wear 3–4 times a day for 30–45 min sessions as needed.
- A full extension resting pan splint is fitted to wear approximately 3 times a day to minimize extensor lags at the MP level.
- Functional electrical stimulation (FES) may be used PRN to enhance tendon excursion within 48 h postoperatively.

S.F.M. Duncan and C.W. Flowers, *Therapy of the Hand and Upper Extremity: Rehabilitation Protocols*, DOI 10.1007/978-3-319-14412-2_101, © Springer International Publishing Switzerland 2015

4 Weeks

- As possible, it is important to begin reducing the wearing time with the various splints. This will include both the dynamic flexion and extension splints.
- Progressive strengthening may be initiated, so long as the patient's hand has minimal edema.

6–8 Weeks

- It is important to begin weaning the patient out of the extension splint at this time if not attempted earlier.

Discharge Criteria

- Patient should be independent in all self-care activities and have begun return to light household activities.

Note: The initial AROM and PROM obtained in surgery should be recorded. It is also important to be informed of the quality of the extensor tendon(s) at the time of surgery.

Chapter 102
FCU to EDC, FDS (Ring) to EDC, OR PT to EDC Tendon Transfers

2 Weeks

- The bulky compressive dressing is removed and appropriate edema control is initiated as necessary.
- A wrist and MP flexion block splint is fitted positioning the wrist in 30° of extension and the MP joints in 0–10° of flexion for continual wear. If extensor lags are present at the PIP joint level, a full extension resting pan splint may be fitted in place of the wrist and MP flexion block.

4–4½ Weeks

- AROM exercises are initiated to the digits and to the wrist for 10 min sessions each hour. Tendon transfer exercises are initiated as follows:

  o FCU to EDC: active flexion and ulnar deviation of the wrist is attempted along with simultaneous extension of the digits.

  o PT to EDC: Active pronation of the forearm is attempted along with simultaneous extension of the digits.

  o FDS to EDC: Active flexion of the IP joints is attempted simultaneously with extension of the MP joints (claw exercise).

S.F.M. Duncan and C.W. Flowers, *Therapy of the Hand and Upper Extremity: Rehabilitation Protocols*, DOI 10.1007/978-3-319-14412-2_102,
© Springer International Publishing Switzerland 2015

- The PIP and DIP joints may be taped in flexion to facilitate excursion of the EDC at the MP joint level while exercising.
- EMG biofeedback may be used as necessary to facilitate muscle reeducation.
- Scar management techniques such as scar massage with lotion and the use of otoform or elastomer are initiated to remodel the subcutaneous adhesions and cutaneous scar.
- FES may be initiated to enhance muscle reeducation and tendon excursion.
- The wrist and MP flexion block splint is continued between exercise sessions and at night.

6 Weeks

- PROM exercises may be initiated to increase passive flexion of the digits.
- Since extrinsic extensor tightness is common at this point, it is important to not only perform passive flexion to the digits but simultaneously to the wrist as well.
- Taping and/or dynamic flexion splinting may be initiated as needed to resolve joint and/or tendon tightness.

Note: It is important to be watchful for the development of extensor lags at the MP level and adjust the therapy accordingly.

- Extension splinting is continued between exercise sessions and at night. Frequently, patients are fitted with a long dorsal outrigger to wear during the day in place of a long static splint to maintain excursion of the EDC and yet allow the patient more normal use of the hand.
- Progressive strengthening may be initiated.

Additional Comments

- Initiation of PROM and/or dynamic flexion splinting should be delayed if there are extensor lags $\geq 30°$. With such extensor lags muscle stimulation and extension splinting should be emphasized along with extension exercises.

Discharge Criteria

- Patient should be able to independently perform all self-care activities.

Chapter 103
Flexor Tendon Repair: Early Mobilization (Zones 1–3)

0–5 Days

- Continue bulky compressive dressing.

3–5 Days

- The bulky dressing is removed.
- A light compressive dressing is applied for edema control.
- A full dorsal blocking splint (DBS) is fitted to the wrist and digits for continual wear with the wrist at 20° of flexion, MCPs at 50° of flexion, and IPs at full extension.
- Controlled passive mobilization is initiated every hour (Modified Duran Program) within restraints of the DBS as stated in the handout "Home Exercise Program for Flexor Tendon Repairs (Initial 4½ weeks)."
- Patient is not permitted any use of hand for daily activities.

2 Weeks

- Initiate scar management techniques.

3½ Weeks

- Begin AROM slowly within the constraints of the splint, making a fist and straightening the fingers—25 repetitions.

S.F.M. Duncan and C.W. Flowers, *Therapy of the Hand and Upper Extremity: Rehabilitation Protocols*, DOI 10.1007/978-3-319-14412-2_103, © Springer International Publishing Switzerland 2015

- Provide home program handout "Home Exercise Program for Flexor Tendon Repairs (Initial 4½ weeks)."

4½ Weeks

- The DBS splint is removed every hour for AROM exercises as stated in the handout. Continue with PROM in DBS.
- The splint is continued between exercises and at night.

5 Weeks

- FES may be initiated to flexors.

5½ Weeks

- The DBS is discontinued.
- An extension splint is fitted to wear between exercises and at night. This should be fitted to the patient's active extension. DO NOT do passive extension.
- Active exercises are performed hourly as stated in the handout (5½ weeks postoperatively).
- Begin light pickups with hand. You may begin light use of hand for bathing.

6 Weeks

- Passive extension exercises are initiated to the wrist and digits.
- Hand may be used as an assist in dressing, bathing, and light hygiene.

8 Weeks

- Strengthening is initiated with putty and hand helper. Light grasp is allowed.
- No lifting or heavy use of the hand is allowed.
- Patient may eat with hand, lift small glass, and increase activities.

10–12 Weeks

- May return to full use of the hand.

***Note*: If the patient has an associated digital nerve repair in which the repair is under some degree of tension, the patient should be fitted with a separate digital DBS in 30° of PIP joint flexion. This splint is progressively straightened by 10° starting at the third week.

Discharge Criteria

- Patient will be independent in all self-care activities and eating.

Chapter 104
Flexor Tendon Repair: Delayed Mobilization (Zones 1–5)

0–3 Weeks

- Bulky compressive dressing.

3 Weeks

- The bulky dressing is removed.
- Edema control is applied PRN.
- A dorsal blocking splint is fitted to the wrist and digits for continual wear with the wrist at 30° of flexion, MCPs at 50° of flexion, and IPs in full extension.
- Active and passive ROM exercises are initiated within the splint in 15 min/h.
- Blocking exercises to the PIP joints may be included.
- Scar management techniques may be initiated.
- Patient is not permitted any use of hand for daily activities.

4½ Weeks

- Active ROM to the digits and wrist are initiated out of the splint.
- The splint is continued between exercises and at night.
- FES may be used to increase tendon excursion.
- Begin light eating activities and use hand as assist in bathing.

S.F.M. Duncan and C.W. Flowers, *Therapy of the Hand and Upper Extremity: Rehabilitation Protocols*, DOI 10.1007/978-3-319-14412-2_104, © Springer International Publishing Switzerland 2015

6 Weeks

- The DBS is discontinued.
- Passive extension exercises are initiated to the wrist and digits.
- An extension splint is fitted to resolve any extrinsic flexor tightness.
- No heavy lifting or use of the hand is allowed.
- Patient may use hand as assist in dressing and hygiene.

8 Weeks

- Progressive strengthening is initiated with putty and hand helper.
- Patient may use hand in progressive resistive activities.

10–12 Weeks

- Return to full use of hand.

Discharge Criteria

- Patient is independent in all self-care activities and may begin light use in household activities.

Chapter 105
Flexor Tenosynovectomy

Day 1

- The bulky dressing is removed.
- Appropriate edema control is applied.
- Active and passive ROM exercises are initiated 15 min/h.
- A safe position splint or a wrist splint is fitted for between exercises.
- Dynamic flexion splinting may be initiated PRN.
- Functional electrical stimulation (FES) may be initiated within 48 h postoperatively to facilitate tendon excursion.

2 Weeks

- Initiate scar management after suture removal.
- Patient can begin eating, light dressing, and bathing activities.

4–6 Weeks

- Gentle, progressive strengthening is initiated.
- Patient should be able to feed self, dress independently, and bathe.

***Note*: As ROM exercises are initiated it is very important to emphasize isolated blocking exercises to the PIP and DIP joints, as well as differential tendon gliding exercises in order to maximize and optimize restoration of digital flexion.

S.F.M. Duncan and C.W. Flowers, *Therapy of the Hand and Upper Extremity: Rehabilitation Protocols*, DOI 10.1007/978-3-319-14412-2_105,
© Springer International Publishing Switzerland 2015

Discharge Criteria

• Patient will be independent in all self-care activities progressing to moderate housekeeping activities.

Chapter 106
Tendon Transfers to Finger Flexors

3 Weeks

- The bulky dressing is removed and edema control is initiated as needed.
- A dorsal blocking splint is fitted positioning the wrist in 20° of flexion, the MP joints in 50° of flexion, and the PIP and DIP joints in neutral for continual wear.
- Active and passive ROM exercises are initiated within the restraint of the splint for 10 min sessions each hour throughout the course of the day. Exercises place emphasis on blocking to maximize excursion of the long flexors.
- FES (Functional electrical stimulator) may be initiated for muscle reeducation and to facilitate proximal excursion of the long flexors. With these tendon transfers the negative (active electrode) is placed either over the radial nerve along the humeral level or over the muscle belly of the ECRL and the positive electrode (indifferent electrode) is placed along the radial side of the forearm in midlateral position.
- Scar management techniques including scar retraction, scar massage with lotion, and the use of otoform is initiated.

S.F.M. Duncan and C.W. Flowers, *Therapy of the Hand and Upper Extremity: Rehabilitation Protocols*,
DOI 10.1007/978-3-319-14412-2_106,
© Springer International Publishing Switzerland 2015

6 Weeks

- The dorsal blocking splint is discontinued.
- Active and gentle passive ROM exercises are initiated in extension for the wrist and digits. Tendon transfer exercises are emphasized by attempting radial wrist extension while simultaneously attempting to make a fist.
- An extension resting pain splint is fitted to wear between exercise sessions and at night to resolve any extrinsic extensor tightness which may have developed.
- All extension splinting along with passive extension is performed in a gradual and progressive manner to prevent stretching out the transfer.

8 Weeks

- Progressive strengthening may be initiated with a nerf ball and progressing to a hand exerciser.
- Extension splinting is discontinued.

Discharge Criteria

- Patient should be able to independently perform all self-care activities.

Chapter 107
Zancolli Lasso

3–5 Days

- The bulky compressive dressing is removed and a light compressive dressing is applied as needed.
- A dorsal blocking splint is fitted positioning the wrist in $0°$ of flexion with the MPs in $50°$ of flexion and the IPs in neutral position for continual wear.
- Active and passive ROM exercises are initiated to the digits within the restraints of the dorsal blocking splint for 10 min sessions each hour.
- Patient may complete light pickups within the constraints of the splint.

2 Weeks

- Initiate scar management.

3 Weeks

- FES (Functional electrical stimulator) may be initiated to enhance the excursion of the long finger flexors.

6 Weeks

- The dorsal blocking splint may be reduced to an MP extension splint with a well-molded palmar bar. The purpose of the palmar bar is to prevent the MPs from "popping out" or fully extending within the restraints of the MP block splint.

S.F.M. Duncan and C.W. Flowers, *Therapy of the Hand and Upper Extremity: Rehabilitation Protocols*,
DOI 10.1007/978-3-319-14412-2_107,
© Springer International Publishing Switzerland 2015

- Active and passive ROM exercises may be initiated to the wrist.
- Patient may use hand for dressing, eating, and hygiene within the constraints of the splint.

8–10 Weeks

- In most cases the MP extension block splint maybe discontinued. It is important to monitor MP extension at this time. If the patient is able to achieve full active extension at the MP level and tends to hyperextend the MP extension block should be continued for an additional 3 weeks.
- At this point, the patient may resume normal use of the hand in basically all activities.

Discharge Criteria

- Patient will be able to dress, bathe, eat, and complete light hygiene activities independently.

Index

S.F.M. Duncan and C.W. Flowers, *Therapy of the Hand and Upper Extremity: Rehabilitation Protocols*, DOI 10.1007/978-3-319-14412-2, © Springer International Publishing Switzerland 2015